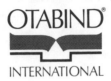
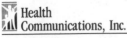

Kind Words For Caring People

Daily Affirmations For Caregivers

Sefra Kobrin Pitzele

Health Communications, Inc.
Deerfield Beach, Florida

©1993 Sefra Kobrin Pitzele
ISBN 1-55874-210-7

Publisher: Health Communications, Inc.
          3201 S.W. 15th Street
          Deerfield Beach, FL 33442-8190

Cover Design by Barbara Bergman

This book is dedicated with love to my mother, Esther Kobrin, who took loving care of my father, Meyer (Mike) Kobrin, as his precious health and ability diminished in his final years.

To Florence (Flo) Charton, who loved Dave and cared for him with passion and devotion until his last breath.

To Beulah Leiter, whose beloved husband Bob cared for her with great love.

To all caregivers, everywhere, I send a warm hug and a special prayer of thanks for your hard work.

Caregiving is a job that no one applies for, no one expects or wants to do. Whether you are caregiving by choice because you wouldn't have it any other way or by default because if you don't do it, it won't be done, it's one of the most difficult jobs known to humankind. Caregiving is the only job that requires service 24 hours a day, seven days a week.

Even the strongest, the most staunch and most willing will wear out with the effort. Some caregivers know the end result will be the death of the one they love — the disease is terminal. Others, dealing with chronic situations, just don't know what their future holds — whether they are to be caregivers for 20 months or 20 years.

Yes, professionals can be caregivers too, but they get to go home after their shift is over. This in no way diminishes the professional's role but we all know it's the one who lives there, who answers the calls for help in the night, who holds the hand of a suffering loved one, who has the hardest time. Watching those we care for deeply lose their zest for living, their mental or physical ability and seeing the light in their eyes grow dull is sad. Life brings trials and we must face them.

A New Year

The beginning of a whole new year — a year that may be marked with joy or sorrow. A year that might be full of uncertainties or promises for each new day. A year when everything might seem right or might go wrong.

When we were young, we looked at each new year as an adventure, a time to meet other young people and have fun. New Year's meant parties, perhaps shared family traditions and looking forward to yet more fun and growing a bit older.

To face each new year now with a smile may be more difficult. We are unsure of our loved one's health and perhaps our own as well. We are uncertain whether we can continue in this difficult role of caregiver but we know we will because there is no other choice. We move forward to face whatever the year will bring.

. . . .

Taking each day singly, not looking at the greater picture, will help me hold on to my health, my sanity and my dreams.

JANUARY 2
"I Don't Mind"

It seemed to everyone that the situation was getting out of hand. Joanne was so tired she could barely respond when visitors stopped by. "John was up at least 10 times last night. I didn't get much sleep," she explained.

Her husband of 45 years had Alzheimer's disease. With no concept of time, he awoke night after night to wander around the house. Worried that he might hurt himself, she would get up and put him back to bed.

One afternoon, Aggie, a dear friend offered to care for John for a few hours so that Joanne could nap or get out for a while. "Oh no! Thanks so much but I don't mind. He's my responsibility and there is no reason for anyone else to take over." Aggie knew enough to keep quiet but she worried about Joanne's health.

Sometimes the problem is right in front of us and we still can't see or face it. It's okay to let someone help me.

True Love Lasts

Dennis was asked over and over again, "Why do you stay with Bonnie now that her MS is so bad? There can't be much in it for you." Each time someone brought up the issue his answer was the same.

"Bonnie and I married for better or for worse, in sickness and in health and the only thing about Bonnie that has really changed is her physical ability. She is still the wittiest, most loving and charitable woman I've ever met. I would never consider leaving her."

When asked if the physical care he gives her isn't too heavy a burden, Dennis is quick to reply that there are always friends, family members or professional caregivers to help him out. "They all love her, too," he answers with a smile.

. . . .

For some people, giving care to their loved ones comes easily. I know I have the emotional and physical strength to continue loving and caring for my loved one even though it does get hard sometimes.

JANURY 4

Change

As we grow older we change; it's inevitable. We don't look or act at 60 the way we did at 16 and few of us would want to! Like everything else in life, change can be easy or very difficult.

We never expected that someone we care about deeply would become mentally or physically ill. And we certainly never expected to be that person's primary caregiver. But when circumstances change and illness enters our lives, we have only two choices.

The first is to stay and take the good with the bad. The second, of course, is to leave or not to accept the responsibility. Caregiving needs come at all levels, from merely helping with bathing and dressing all the way to full care. By looking for the best solutions and getting help when necessary, many of us can choose to stay.

....

I don't like the situation we are in but I respect myself and the one I care for enough to handle our problem in an adult way.

Anger

In the beginning, caregiving often just creeps up. One day we see that the person we love is less and less competent and that we have taken over most of the chores.

In many cases, this need progresses and we soon are doing the other's personal care as well as our own. Often we become sleep-deprived, our energy wanes and we may develop health problems of our own. After all, one's body can only take so much.

Without any respite, caregiving can be a 24-hour-a-day job. It is not uncommon for anger to set in — anger at our situation, anger at what has happened to a person we love and anger at feeling trapped. To our dismay, we may also feel angry at the one who is sick, yet we really understand there is no one to blame. Illness just happens. No one plans it.

....

Anger is a normal emotion and I can find some appropriate ways to vent my feelings.

JANUARY 6
Home Alone

Many caregivers need to hold down jobs in order to pay the rent and put groceries on the table. More often than not, at the beginning of a chronic or even a terminal illness, it is safe for the care recipient to stay home alone.

As the months and years pass, however, we recognize signs of danger. Perhaps medicines were forgotten during the day or the lunch we left in the refrigerator was not eaten. If we have a night job, we may find clues that the person has wandered around the house.

At this juncture there is a very difficult decision to make. We could quit work, possibly retire or go on welfare to stay home and caregive or we may try to hire help or solicit county assistance. Visiting nurses and home health aides might be the answer.

....

I have to work or we will lose our home and our car and won't be able to pay our bills. With innovation and perseverance I will make sure a program is in place so I can continue to work.

Daycare

Sometimes serious problems surface when a caregiver needs to work or perhaps is trying to do all the caregiving alone. One solution might be to place the person we are caring for in a good adult daycare program.

At first we may feel disappointed that we can't do it all. But eventually we may see that our loved one is happier.

We had not considered that he or she might be bored and lonely, losing interpersonal and practical skills due to lack of stimulation from others. Daycare can be an ideal situation for both the sick person and the caregiver.

. . . .

A certified, safe and stimulating daycare program will put me at ease and we will both be happier.

JANUARY 8
Failing Health

No job requires more time, energy or personal devotion than caregiving. Whether given willingly or begrudgingly, caregiving — especially if complete caregiving is needed — can take a terrible toll on the health of the person giving the care.

Elderly women with medical problems of their own, such as heart disease or arthritis, for example, might find their own illness escalating in the face of too little sleep and too few moments of relief.

Sometimes our bodies know us better than we think and the caregiver eventually becomes so ill that hospitalization or serious medical intervention is needed. Only then do we realize that we must accept help — that no one person can do it all alone.

....

It took serious illness for me to recognize my limitations. I understand now that I must get help or both of us will need caregivers.

Not Forever

Mention stroke or a broken hip and what automatically comes to mind is a nursing home. In fact, that may be where the sick person ends up — but perhaps only for the recovery period.

Nursing homes are often used these days instead of a long hospital stay. Patients enter for the duration of their healing process and then are released to go home or to a relative's house.

Certainly the underlying medical problems remain and caregiving at home is still required but the immediate crisis is over and the patient is back home where, at least for now, he belongs.

. . . .

My loved one belongs at home with me. For now, at least, I can continue to give care in our home.

Childlike Behavior

Perhaps the saddest and hardest kind of caregiving is needed when a person we love dearly — husband, wife, mother, father — suffers atrophy of the brain due to accident, injury or a disease such as Alzheimer's.

Suddenly the body is there but the person we knew who inhabited it is gone for good. Just reconciling ourselves to that fact is most difficult. Taking care of a childlike adult takes a tremedous toll on us emotionally.

....

In order to give good care — warm and loving care — I must separate my old memories from the reality of today.

Grieving

How sad the day is when we finally realize that the person who has had a stroke has healed as much as they are able, when the person who has multiple sclerosis must now stay in bed most of the day.

Our need to grieve may never even occur to us for we are too busy caring for them and, barely for ourselves. Not surprisingly, grief does creep in — sometimes silently — sometimes causing great emotional upheaval.

We may deny and deny, but reality — truth — finally is seen. Not surprisingly, some of us buckle under the added weight of grief. This is normal and to be expected, yet a terribly sad experience.

....

I must allow myself the right to grieve —
for all that used to be — for all we will
be deprived of in the future — so I can go
on to do what must be done.

Two-Way Response

In many instances, constant and complete caregiving is needed for someone who is quite incapacitated, but just as often, only ongoing assistance is required to maintain the status quo, perhaps help getting into and out of the bath and bed and some assistance with food preparation.

Such a person may be quite capable of maintaining relationships, not only with friends and family but with a husband or wife as well. This is crucial when the caregiver and the one accepting care are married. It's all too easy to lose sight of the relationship in the face of long-term illness or disability.

Never losing sight of the fact that we are giving care to someone we love dearly and who loves us allows us both to maintain dignity, individuality and any expression of love we wish to demonstrate to each other.

....

Because of illness, I tend to forget how life used to be. If we both work hard together, we can maintain our deep love.

JANUARY 13
Privacy

Needing another person's help to take care of personal needs can — to say the least — be overwhelming. Some care recipients are degraded by a complete lack of privacy.

Fearing that a loved one will hurt himself, some caregivers, without even asking for it, take that individual's right to privacy. They hover in the bathroom, kitchen or bedroom, generally shadowing the sick person's every move — a bit too conscientiously.

Ill people deserve privacy and time to be alone — as long as they are safe. Time spent simply looking out the window or sitting alone in the bathroom is extremely important for both personal dignity and privacy.

I must struggle to remember to treat my loved one as I would wish to be treated and never to take away basic human rights.

JANURY 14

More Privacy

The other side of the privacy issue is that many caregivers, besides enduring the emotional and physical strain, silently lament their own lack of privacy.

It seems that the sick person is always hovering, always needing something, always there, invading what precious time the caregiver has. It hurts not to have any time alone, away from the rigors of caregiving, but it also makes me feel guilty for wanting it.

There are solutions for this problem: talking with the recipient, if that person is capable of understanding, and asking for some time alone, or asking a relative or neighbor to relieve us for a couple of hours a week so we can have some free time.

....

I feel guilty that I resent giving care to my loved one but I know I should take care of my own needs as well. From this day forward I shall try to meet that goal.

Bartering

The demands that caregiving puts on us are not unlike those we had as parents of a new baby — just as we think we can settle down for a while, our attention is needed. But now we care for a fully grown incapacitated person.

Few of us have forgotten how we stumbled through life in those early parenting days. Now we are most likely 40 or more years older, trying to perform an even more demanding job with no respite.

There are practical solutions — having our loved one participate in an adult daycare program, hiring help or bartering with a friend or neighbor for a few hours off in exchange for baking a couple of pies or darning some socks. We won't know unless we ask, what some good friends or neighbor might be willing to do.

. . . .

Ask. This is the key. I will learn to ask for help so I can stay healthy and continue to care for my loved one.

JANUARY 16

Alternatives

Most of us think about what will happen when we can no longer take care of ourselves. Some people tell their children, "Anything but a nursing home. Promise me you won't do that to me."

For some, a nursing home is the only answer. But there are alternatives for those times when we need to be relieved of full-time caregiving.

Respite care is available in many areas where a medical facility can be used while we vacation or recover from an operation or injury. There are group homes for senior adults which may be a fine choice. Share-a-home situations proliferate where a young, healthy person — often a student — exchanges room and board for doing inside and outside chores. Personal care attendants can be hired as well.

....

I honor my own human needs. I need not feel guilty if I cannot always be the one to give care.

Leaving

Sarah was furious. For all those years, 35 of them, she stuck by the old coot, both on and off the wagon. The only reason she did was that between drinking spells he was a fair husband — he brought home a little money and was kind to her and the kids.

But things were different now. He'd been drinking steadily for five years and going downhill all the while. Now he'd had a stroke which left him completely impaired. The doctor was discussing his discharge to go home — with Sarah to care for him.

"I am not taking this drunk home. Put him in a nursing home or anywhere you want. I've devoted too much time to him already. I'm only 53 and I have never had a life. Now it's my turn and I'm getting a divorce. He's history in my life."

. . . .

Wanting my own life may sound selfish, but I have the right to choose and I choose personal freedom.

Special Children

Caregiving can come gradually, with illness taking over slowly, or suddenly, after a stroke or an accident.

But for those who have a tiny bundle placed in their arms, their newborn babe, and are told that this child will need care for life, caregiving comes suddenly, at a time when it is least expected. It is frightening, overwhelming.

Severely handicapped children used to be "put away" — the parents advised to forget they were born. Nowadays most people take such a child home and begin, day by day, to deal with the problems they will face for the rest of the child's life.

. . . .

Caring for a special needs child is difficult but we love this child and he adds joy to our lives daily. We would not consider letting anyone else care for him, especially away from us.

Laughter

Sid and Jill were laughing again. They always had so much fun together. They had always been able to use humor in an emotional crisis, an uncanny ability to see the flip side of a problem.

Jill was helping Sid in the shower, as she had since a stroke left him impaired on his left side. The soap slid out of his hand over and over and she retrieved it each time, getting soaked. Finally she stripped, got in the shower and they both got clean.

"As long as we're here, Sweetie, how about a hug?" said Sid with glinting eyes and a great big smile. Sid and Jill never lost their love for each other, both physical and emotional, and never passed up a chance for laughter and closeness.

"You bet, Toots!" She smiled as his good arm encircled her.

....

What was good before has become wonderful now as daily we create new memories to cherish. We are so blessed.

JANURARY 20

Doing Too Much

We want to do everything we can to help someone we love who needs caregiving whether a parent, a sibling or a spouse.

In fact, some of us have a tendency to give a bit too much, to forget that the other person still has rights and needs. In one case, for example, a woman helped her father dress and undress and sat in the bathroom while he took a bath.

Finally he said, "Honey, I don't know how to say this without hurting you but you are doing too much. Please let me put on what clothes I can and check on me once in a while in the tub. I know how much you care but even sick I deserve respect and privacy."

....

I know now that caregiving doesn't always mean taking over. I didn't consider his rights. From now on I will never forget.

Still Caregiving

Some people assume that when a spouse or parent is placed in a nursing home their role as caregiver is over. Nothing could be further from the truth.

Nursing homes can't do everything. As excellent as many are, they can't love each patient or go on shopping trips to buy new clothing as the old wears out. Nursing homes don't bake chocolate chip cookies and they don't take people home for a holiday meal.

Certainly, placement in a nursing home is necessary in many instances to provide safety and care when that cannot be done adequately at home. The caregiver finally has some time to be alone, or with friends and family, to take care of long overdue problems but their care is still needed for many things.

....

I feel both guilt and relief now that my spouse is in a nursing home but now I understand that the caregiving goes on — in a different way.

JANUARY 22
Enabling

There is another kind of caregiving, one which is not good for either party, yet neither knows how to stop it. Both are trapped in a behavior pattern that is called enabling. One person demonstrates unacceptable behavior, such as drinking or drug use, while the other carefully covers up the tracks and protects them.

Enabling is a negative type of caregiving. The enabler is always on the watch to make life easier, to make sure the job, church or community doesn't know what is happening behind closed doors.

Enablers need psychological help for they cannot get out of their situation unless they do some hard work with regard to their own needs and habits and discover why they need to sanction unacceptable behavior. Help is available from many sources.

....

I spent 10 years enabling and two learning why. I am free now to live as I choose without having to take care of everyone else's needs.

This Is Hard

Herm really loved his wife — at least he did during all the years when she was well. He didn't know how he felt now. These days he was tired beyond describing. Caregiving was hard for him and he himself wasn't all that well. His wife just wasn't the same anymore.

Every time a friend or family member called he sounded more down and more fatigued but when they asked if he was all right, he quickly popped back with, "Sure. We're both fine. I can handle this easily." But those who knew him well were very, very worried.

One day his daughter stopped by and found Herm in tears — uncontrollable sobs. He could take no more. He collapsed. He was hospitalized for complete exhaustion and depression and his wife was cared for by the family until he was better. Afterwards they saw to it that he got help and relief.

. . . .

It took a complete collapse for me to understand that no one person can do it all. It's okay for me to need help and to ask for it.

23

The Vacation

For years the couple had talked about driving to the West Coast on a vacation as soon as they both retired. Their dream trip was all planned when they were in an auto accident. Both had injuries but the husband was seriously injured, losing both legs.

Family and friends immediately rallied to help in any way they could. There was so much the couple were mourning, from the loss of his legs to giving up their dream vacation. A year passed and both recovered, although he was now in a wheelchair.

What they didn't know was that their oldest child and her husband had secretly planned that her parents would still get to go west, with the young couple going along for assistance and sharing of joys and problems. How wonderful!

....

A serious injury brought us even closer as a family. We still have each other and we have now had the joy of fulfilling our life's dream as well.

Pent-Up Anger

Fatigue is a well-known part of being a care-giver, yet other elements enter the picture as well. For some there is a new closeness between caregiver and receiver. Others share laughter more often.

After months or years of caregiving, pent-up anger and frustration may reach a boiling point and we find ourselves yelling in frustration at the other person, who doesn't understand the reasons for our anger and frustration. Sometimes the ill person is verbally abused or even beaten.

There are ways to get help and some relief from our difficult situation. Social service agencies can send in a caregiver for a few hours each week. Some communities provide art programs or daycare.

....

There is always a better solution than showing my anger to one I love. I didn't know I could ask for help but now that I do, I will ask when my anger and frustration build up.

Just Today

When an individual who used to be intelligent and respected suddenly becomes childlike, we may not know how to treat that person. We were equals and now this person functions like a recalcitrant three-year-old.

There is the clue — dealing with the person as though he were three years old, in an adult tone and with definite respect for the individual and his rights — without ever losing sight of his emotional fragility.

By speaking gently and quietly, giving instructions with assistance, one thing at a time, and by not projecting or planning more than an hour or so ahead, we can care for that person with as little confusion as possible as we move through each day.

....

It is very difficult for me to treat an adult like a child but I understand why. I'm angry about it and it's hard but it's all right for me to own my feelings.

Inaccessible Places

From the time Judy developed multiple sclerosis she feared going into a wheelchair and prayed she would never have to. Now she was in an electric chair, complete with every gadget available. Surprisingly she was relieved, for she had more energy to spend each day now that she was not struggling so hard to walk.

Her husband was pleased that she felt less pain and fatigue and they decided to attend the theater, a favorite pastime. Tickets bought, a good dinner in their bellies, they got to the theater only to find it was not wheelchair accessible.

Sadly they turned away, were given a refund for their tickets and started home. "Boy, we really learned a lesson tonight. Never assume a place is wheelchair accessible. We'll have to call ahead and ask every time we leave the house."

....

We will continue to do what we choose but we will have to plan ahead to make sure the way is clear to accommodate my wheelchair.

27

JANUARY 28
Going Out To Dinner

Harriet and Don loved to go out to eat — at least they loved it until she had a stroke, but now, with her right side badly affected, going out was almost impossible.

It wasn't really impossible but, in truth, Don was embarrassed by Harriet's handicap. She made so much noise eating and dropped so much food trying to feed herself that he felt everyone was staring at them.

One day he confided his feelings to a friend at the "stroke group" he attended every Tuesday evening. "Heavens," said the friend, "the same thing happened to us. Call ahead and ask to be seated a bit away from the main room. Then go very early, like 4:30 or 5:00, when few people are dining. Cut up her food and offer to feed her and both of you can enjoy eating out again, just like us!"

....

Every day I learn new ways to deal with my wife's handicap. By being open about our problems, I find people are willing to share their successes with me.

Not By Choice

When we are put in the position of giving care to a person we love deeply, we can expect our lives to change — sometimes drastically. The first, and seemingly the most important decision, is to decide who will do the caregiving.

Sometimes the choice is obvious if the person is married or living in a home with family members, as long as they are physically and mentally capable of taking on the job — and a job it is — 24 hours a day of devotion, love, strength and care.

At first, caregiving may feel awkward because, as with any new job, it is unclear what it really entails. As the days pass we find out, by need, by accident, by hook or by crook. Including the care recipient in our decision-making process, if possible, will help.

. . . .

Feeling my way into the caregiving process was not easy at first but now I understand my new role and am working hard to adjust.

Making Love

For six decades Shirley and Rob were a cohesive unit and everyone who knew them envied their relationship. It was relatively rare for him to be seen without her or vice-versa. Their life was filled with grandchildren and volunteer work.

Then Shirley developed brain atrophy and her personality underwent a radical change. She became combative and nasty. Rob was confused until the doctor explained.

He could take care of her physically but she wanted him to make love to her, often mentioning it even in public. He was so embarrassed. "How can I make love to a person I don't even know? She's a total stranger! I hate this."

When our loved one expects everything to stay the same even when it is all different, real problems can ensue.

....

Saying no to my wife is one of the hardest things I've ever done but I know it's all right in order to maintain my own self-worth.

Keeping A Chart

Most of us remember when we were children and had a personal problem, our parents or counselor might suggest we make a Positive-Negative chart listing all the good and bad or difficult factors, to help us with decision-making. This is a good idea when caregiving gets to be too much to handle.

The list might also include suggestions such as "Need help with bathing," or "Can't do own grocery shopping — need someone to do it for us." Looking at our problems in black and white allows more objectivity.

Finding assistance in the areas where we need it is hard but the physician, social agencies and family and friends are there to help with solutions that we might not have thought of.

. . . .

At first I was overwhelmed by sadness and guilt that I could not do it all. Now I am so grateful that I learned to ask for help.

FEBRUARY 1

A Sense Of Duty

Some people choose to be caregivers out of a sense of duty. This was the case with Karl, who had just received a divorce from Anna, his wife of 15 years. They had always put up a good front in public but he was fed up with her when he discovered she was using drugs on the sly.

Ten days after their divorce she had a devastating stroke. They had promised each other that neither would ever go to a nursing home and he felt obligated to take on her care. To everyone's surprise, he brought her to their old home.

Family and friends were dismayed at his decision. But he stood by her and gave her care for three years until another stroke took her life. "It was my duty. She had no one else to help. I would not have done it any other way."

I am not sorry that I helped a person whom I once loved dearly. First of all, I must be able to respect myself.

A Topsy-Turvy World

Linda had always taken care of other people, not because she had to but because she chose to. As a nurse she was well-liked and she particularly enjoyed working in intensive care or the emergency room.

She loved going to work each day and was a very happy person . . . until her mother had a stroke. Then Linda's world turned topsy-turvy. She and her husband converted the dining room into a bedroom, put in a hospital bed and brought her mother home. Linda left work every day knowing that her mother would need more care and she gave it, willingly.

After a weight loss she couldn't afford, Linda went to her doctor, who told her, "Linda, you must get help to care for your mother. In order to reserve some energy for your husband and children, you must take care of yourself first."

. . . .

I've never let myself be first in anything but I now understand that if I don't, there won't be anything left for my family.

33

FEBRUARY 3
Time Out

Many parents deal with their young children's small infractions by giving them a Time Out. As adults we sometimes call Time Out when we are about to explode with anger and we go for a walk or take a nice bath until we cool off.

Now that we are caregivers, Time Out takes on a whole new meaning. Caregivers have a tendency to forget their own needs or they won't even recognize that they have any. But it is imperative to take time out at least once each week, just for ourselves.

Additionally, going on a short vacation, even if it's just to a hotel in our own city, will give us renewed energy and a new perspective on our caregiving process. Everyone needs at least a small amount of time out.

....

It seems so selfish to take time away from the person who needs me most but when I consider what would happen if I couldn't give care, I realize the importance of getting away.

Sharing

Not everyone is physically, psychologically, emotionally or even practically equipped to be a full-time caregiver. When this is the case, family or professional help should be called upon for assistance. A good example is when the caregiver's health is not good and help is needed just to get by.

By tapping into resources available in the family or from social services in the form of visiting nurses and home health aides, most of us can find some way to set up a plan to share the burden of caregiving.

This is easier said than done, for while we may intellectually understand the need for help, sometimes it is emotionally difficult to follow through with a plan.

. . . .

By letting someone else do some of the caregiving I have given a gift both to myself and to my beloved.

Suicide

Some kinds of caregiving are much harder than others. Watching over a person who is suicidal is one of the hardest of all. Anyone who has done this knows how heartrending it is.

This type of caregiving should only be undertaken in an emergency situation, for example, while waiting for medical help to arrive or perhaps waiting until a newly prescribed medication takes effect.

In most cases, a person who is really suicidal should be temporarily hospitalized. The terror of knowing that someone we love deeply could harm themselves makes us keep our eyes on them every instant until help arrives. No one should have to do this kind of caregiving for more than a few days.

. . . .

Whether the person is a teenager or an elderly adult, any suggestion of suicide should always be taken seriously and acted upon.

Roles

There is no situation in which family roles can change faster than when a family member becomes incapacitated by illness or injury.

The child who is the class clown may sit hour after hour at the sick person's bedside, while Aunt Marie may appoint herself chief cook. People who have run away from their problems might come back to roost, while the most stable might not be able to give any care at all.

There is no way to judge ahead of time. If the situation is likely to become long-term, a family council is appropriate. Deciding which role each person will take and what they will be responsible for helps lighten the load of the primary caregiver. All the secondary caregivers — family and friends — can then still have plenty of time to pursue their personal interests as well.

. . . .

Treating our loved one's need for caregiving as a family problem and sharing the responsibility will help and be better for all of us.

37

Resources

A multitude of resources is available these days to assist caregivers. Caregivers frequently feel isolated but this need not be the case. All we have to do is reach out and pick up the phone.

From Meals On Wheels to help with keeping the home clean, to telephone support or check-in services — help abounds in most communities. Some churches send out "Befrienders" while other groups have different programs which include visiting.

Congregate dining activities are found nearly everywhere now and chore services are springing up. Daycare services and other programs proliferate and in special instances there is adult foster care for help on a temporary basis.

....

It seems that everyone is trying to help. All I need do is reach out and ask. This way I can still be effective in my caregiving role.

The Money Problem

One of the biggest problems that arises when we are thrust into the role of caregiver is the loss or potential loss of income. We might have to give up our job or change our hours. The person who needs care has suddenly had to quit working.

As hard as it is to keep practical considerations uppermost in mind when we see a loved one going downhill, it is essential to our feeling of security and well-being. Until we handle the financial end of things, we may not be able to settle into our new role.

Looking carefully at lost income or fixed income, perhaps at the cost of modifying a home to make things more accessible, considering what will happen to our benefit or pension program, all this is, unfortunately, part of the reality of being a full-time caregiver.

....

These difficult problems are part of my new role. I can face head on all the difficulties and find the best solutions for us.

FEBRUARY 9
Spirituality

It's interesting that some caregivers who will not leave their loved one for any other reason still find a way to get to their church or synagogue, while others who used to go all the time won't leave for even a few moments.

Many feel distressed that they are no longer attending services, for they feel comforted when they worship. Many are angry at themselves for having such feelings, at their recipients because they are no longer healthy and at God for letting it happen.

Working our way through grief and anger is not easy. It can be a long and time-consuming task but letting go of anger is essential in order to take care of ourselves and someone else as well.

....

At first I was just plain overwhelmed, then I was overwhelmed with my anger at God. I realize now that both were normal feelings which I needed to experience so I could move on with my life.

Relaxing

Sometimes it's possible to take time out during the day while the person you are caring for is at home with you. When your care recipient is watching television or sleeping is an ideal time.

Get a book from the library and learn guided imagery or relaxation. Both are easy and do give us a crucial break in an otherwise hectic day.

These mini-breaks are sometimes what hold a caregiver together, since few get enough sleep, rest or relaxation. We only need 15 minutes and the only limitation is our imagination.

. . . .

A natural skeptic at first, I was surprised to find how much relief I got from guided imagery and relaxation. For a few moments I can let myself be "gone" from all my problems. It feels wonderful.

FEBRUARY 11
Self-Praise

Never since we had newborns — if we had children — have we had a job that demands as much as being a caregiver. All day, every day, all night, every night, we are on call.

It doesn't matter whether we are giving care lovingly and willingly or because there is no one else to help. We need to remember to feel proud of the job we are doing.

Praising ourself is a wonderful way to bolster a sagging ego. Sometimes we even need to sit down and write out what is going right — not what is going wrong. It's amazing how long the list will grow and how surprised we will be at our success.

. . . .

I have to admit that it feels good when I silently praise myself for doing a good job in hard circumstances.

Self-Criticism

Far too many of us have learned to live without getting praise — either as children or as adults. Now that we are in a new kind of job — caregiving — and we are both the boss and all the employees as well, we may find that we are criticizing ourselves.

Phrases such as, "I could have done better" — "I'm not any good at this" — or "I know I'm the only one doing it, but I'm not doing a good enough job" — are fruitless and damage what self-esteem we still have intact.

Learning to say, "I did a good job caregiving today," or "I'm finally learning to read his signals," or even "This was a pretty good day. I kept things going relatively smoothly," are helpful and encourage our self-growth.

. . . .

Self-worth often goes down the drain when we are performing one of life's most difficult jobs — caregiving. I am learning that it feels good to praise myself for a job well done.

Substitutes

For obvious reasons, we don't want to believe that anyone else could take over our job as chief caregiver. Some of us find out when our own health fails or when we need to go into the hospital for surgery or treatment.

Much to our surprise, our care recipient, if he has a brain atrophy disease, may not notice that we were gone. Others may comment favorably on the change, saying, "It was nice to see a new face for a change."

At first we are hurt, we feel pushed aside, no longer important. But once we put this new information in perspective, we recognize that having an alternate caregiver once in a while is an excellent way to get some relief from a tedious job and some time for ourselves.

. . . .

It seemed so self-serving at first to need time just for me when my beloved is so ill but now I understand that getting away for a short time makes me a better caregiver.

In our youth and perhaps during our marriage — when both of us were well — Valentine's Day represented something special. Lucky women could expect flowers, a small gift or perhaps a specially prepared meal.

One woman related this story. His illness made it excruciatingly difficult for her husband to use a pen or pencil. He had persuaded his daytime caregiver (the wife worked) to take him out to buy a card. Just for this she was moved, for he wasn't always in touch with reality.

That evening when she emptied the trash, she found dozens of wrinkled pieces of paper. Each had different words of his love for her but none was complete. He must have worked all day but couldn't write a whole love message. She sat down and cried — for all his past love, for love lost to illness and for her own sadness.

....

Having a person you love be there but not the same as they used to be is so hard. I am adjusting slowly and I will be okay.

FEBRUARY 15

Closeness

Some lucky couples find that the experience of caregiving brings them much closer. This, of course, can only happen when the care recipient is able to communicate thoughts and feelings and, in the best way possible, to demonstrate those feelings.

Pete mentioned that he and Jessy were both happy in their marriage but once he was in a wheelchair they began to really look for even more common interests. Not surprisingly, they found many things to share.

Developing new hobbies and interests and the ability to talk about feelings are among the bonuses caregivers and recipients can share, as well as showing commitment to each other by staying together and really living.

. . . .

I admit that being forced to spend time together made us take a close look at our "happiness." We were always happy, but now we really share our lives.

Details

Molly was always a stickler for details. Everyone knew she had the cleanest house, impeccably neat closets and she cooked outstanding gourmet meals besides. She had it all together — a rare person.

When her mother became ill with Parkinson's disease and moved in with Molly and Bob, Molly expected to take on this new assignment of caregiving with the same aplomb she had always had. She was in for a big surprise.

She hadn't realized how long it would take to keep her mother, who is now somewhat childlike, clean, fed and safe. Molly quickly learned that a casserole is acceptable for dinner and no one ever looks in her dresser drawers. She had to let some aspects of her old life go in order to do the work at hand.

....

Until I let go of my obsessive need to control my environment through cleanliness, I couldn't willingly care for my mother. The job is still hard but I am working hard at making it work.

Limbo

At first, Janice was grateful that Art had not died when they did the emergency surgery on his brain aneurysm. But when he came out of the coma, he was a different person than the husband she had loved.

Since he was unable to care for himself, Janice and the children decided he would go to a nursing home "just for now." She visited him every day and left more depressed each time. Since his face was not changed, she couldn't accept his condition as permanent.

One day she broke into loud, racking sobs. "Why did he live? We all would have been better if he hadn't pulled through. I'm neither a widow nor a divorcee. I'm caught in limbo for all the years he is going to live. It just isn't fair."

....

Life isn't always fair. I knew that in my head but my heart kept overruling my brain. I am adjusting now but I still hate this.

The Chief

Sometimes it is obvious from the beginning and sometimes not until time has passed, but eventually it is apparent to the family that one person alone cannot do all the caregiving.

Giving physical care to another is very hard under the best of circumstances but if the caregiver has some chronic health problem, such as a bad back, it is nearly impossible.

The solution, if there is family, is to have a family council and make assignments to share the responsibility of caregiving. One family member might cook, another shop and yet a third may do the bathing. This way one person is chief caregiver but is surrounded by loving family members sharing the burden.

. . . .

Admitting I couldn't do it all was hard for no one had ever intruded in our life before. But I have learned to accept help so that I too may survive.

So Frightened

The phone rang and he reached out reflexively even though he was upset and didn't want to talk. It was his mother, some 87 years old. "What's wrong, dear? Has anything changed with Darlene?"

She knew him too well, so he told her that Darlene was going downhill fast — it looked like only a few weeks and she would be gone. He sobbed, "How will I live without her, Ma? What will the kids and I do?"

"If I could, I would be there to help, honey. You and the children will need to draw strength from one another. She isn't gone yet and you are frightened of the end. It will take a long time but one day you will be all right again."

. . . .

To watch someone die whom you adore is so awful. I am functioning for my wife and for the children. I know my mother is right and that I will heal in time but it doesn't seem so now.

The Sandwich Generation

Today's caregivers may be in the most unique family situation ever in history. People live longer and couples put off having a family until the wife's career is established — and we have families caring for infants and for grandparents, sometimes under the same roof.

This situation brings with it some unique problems. Young children will have no memories of a healthy grandparent. There are not enough hours in the day and the couple, especially the woman, often gives up something she worked for years to earn, something precious — her profession.

Some grandparents only need minimal care and can function as helpers with the young children. Others need complete care and go to a nursing home, with their family members doing as much as they can on weekends.

....

Each family has to find its own solution, as we did. Board and care worked best for us and I can still work, be a mother and wife and a dutiful, loving daughter.

51

FEBRUARY 21
New Hobbies

How lucky the couple who, despite some need for caregiving, can laugh with each other, be with friends and show they care about each other.

When a person becomes housebound, there are many indoor pastimes that can captivate and entertain them, from stamp collecting to ham radio to doing puzzles together.

When shaking hands keep bridge players from playing, a card rack will let the game go on. When inability to sit for long periods puts the kibosh on board games, crossword puzzles can be fun. There is always a solution if we look hard enough.

. . . .

We were lucky to be able to use illness as a starting place to gain new skills and interests. Life is different now but still great.

Loneliness

In trying to be the perfect caregiver, many of us inadvertently cut ourselves off from our friends and previous activities. Loneliness results, particularly if we are caring for someone who cannot communicate with us.

But we can call and invite close friends in for lunch or perhaps for tea if it's our care recipient's nap time.

Dinner out with friends may be possible, with or without the person we care for. By going out early and not apologizing for the behavior of the individual who is ill, dinner with friends can still be enjoyable.

We can also invite friends in for a potluck or to watch an afternoon football game. People generally don't mind contributing to a meal and helping with clean-up.

....

I am lonely because I have allowed myself to be alone. I need only make some calls to bring family or friends back to our home. I no longer feel ashamed and am willing to reach out.

FEBRUARY 23

Reporting

Not surprisingly, our responsibilities have at least quadrupled. One of the most important is that we must learn how to report changes accurately to our care recipient's physician.

Small changes, such as a two pound weight loss or a slightly diminished appetite, can wait until the next routine doctor's visit. But more important changes — dramatic weight loss, inability to sleep, increased frequency of falling, confusion or medicine side effects — should be reported immediately and accurately.

Be sure to have your pharmacy's and doctor's number and all pertinent information, such as what medicines the person is taking, available at your fingertips. Doctors generally want to know about any major and some minor changes.

. . . .

I hardly have time enough for myself but I understand how important it is to observe and keep track of any significant change with regard to my care recipient.

I Need Help

"Doing the same thing day after day is driving me crazy. Sometimes I feel like hitting my own husband! I can't believe I'm saying this. I'm usually such a gentle person."

Quickly, others in Bianca's support group joined in. "Before I joined the support group, I felt the same way. It isn't that he did anything wrong but that I couldn't stand the sameness, the boredom, each and every day, knowing it would be the same again tomorrow."

Bianca felt a tremendous relief knowing she wasn't the only one who had such thoughts. From that day on she knew there was a group of new friends, people who really understood both her frustration and her joy. Friends made caregiving seem a tiny bit easier.

. . . .

Support groups have offered me so much more than support. They help me maintain my sanity, my sense of humor and my hope.

FEBRUARY 25
....
Belittling

Thelma and Fred had been at each other for years. Even their children didn't pay attention to it any more for they expected the squabbling — it had always been part of their life.

Now that Thelma is in a wheelchair, Fred's nasty remarks and belittling jibes seem to be constant. He has lost sight of what is funny and what is not and uses her handicap to release all his frustration about her injury.

His comments drove all their friends away until Joe finally collared him and gave him a good talking to. "Do you know how small you sound, making fun of your wife? Find a more appropriate way to deal with your frustrations than knocking Thelma or I'm gone too!"

....

Sometimes frustration leads us to say things we don't mean. It took the intervention of a very good friend to help me realize what I was doing. I will never do it again.

Mental Alertness

One of the hardest problems to deal with when we become caregivers is that our lives seem taken over by an invisible enemy we don't know and can barely recognize.

Becoming intellectually stagnant is often an incidental effect of becoming a caregiver but that does not necessarily need to be true. There are all sorts of ways we can keep ourselves current and aware.

Reading the daily newspaper and watching news commentary will help. So will continuing to read. Finding time to be with friends who share stimulating conversation helps immensely. Caregiving plus care receiving need not add up to boredom.

. . . .

Caregiving need not be an isolating, stagnating experience. It takes special effort but I can keep myself intellectually active.

New Education

When a person we care about becomes ill and needs our help, we become almost instant experts on his or her particular disability.

We learn quickly when we understand how important it is to have a full grasp of what is going on in our loved one's body. People who never knew about multiple sclerosis learn in unexpected ways. The families of lupus patients become lupus lay experts.

Doctors appreciate interest and understanding from family members and are generally willing to answer our questions. Most physicians don't mind when we offer up information we have discovered in a magazine or book and ask about it.

. . . .

Families matter tremendously to the wellbeing of the person who needs care. Gathering information and gaining understanding of the illness help us give better and more efficient care.

Hidden Rewards

It is heard time and time again. "We've never been as close as we have since I became ill." Skeptics wonder if this is true because there is no alternative to caregiving. Some also ask if it is really marital closeness or something else, forced by the illness.

If the person who is receiving care is mentally competent, there is no reason to assume this cannot become a personal growth experience for both caregiver and recipient. Like the lady who got a load of lemons and made lemonade, they also can turn a potentially negative situation into a positive one.

Receiving care or giving it need not always herald the ending of a strong marriage. In a strange way the need for caregiving can increase love and redirect caring.

. . . .

I have never thought of caregiving as a burden. Instead, it is just a way I can offer help. I know if the tables were turned, I would receive similar care.

MARCH 1
Time Off

Most people, when they hear the words "respite care" — if they know what it means at all — think of handicapped children. Of course, they are right. Respite care allows parents of mentally or physically handicapped children some time off for a vacation or to handle health problems of their own.

Respite care is available to help other care-givers as well. Many organizations or licensed individuals can provide respite care. Most often the care recipient is placed temporarily in either a facility or a private home.

If we need respite care for health reasons, it may be an absolute necessity. But if it's a vacation we desire or a trip to see a new grandchild, that, too, is just as important. Few caregivers realize how helpful and renewing time away from their problems can be.

....

I felt guilty when I even considered a vacation. But most workers get one each year. Now I understand that taking time away renews me for the next several months.

How frustrating it is for people whose loved ones have Alzheimer's disease. To see someone, once competent, needing care like a small child rips at our hearts.

Yet there are some rewards as well — small rewards. Some of these revolve around reminiscing. Many patients with brain atrophy diseases lose their short-term memory but their long-term memory, for some reason, stays intact, and they love to talk about the past.

Watching grandchildren sit on a grandfather's lap as he points out faces in a photo album from half a century ago, with remarkable accuracy, is terrific. Some people take time to label their photographs for future generations.

Telling about incidents that happened long ago can be taped, for often they are told as if they happened yesterday.

. . . .

With almost every problem in life comes a ray of sunshine. Once I learned to give physical care I could sit back and enjoy reminiscing.

Divorce

Valerie's mother had taken a bad fall and broken her hip and wrist. Naturally Valerie and her husband Todd invited her to recuperate at their home. They didn't know yet that she was falling often and losing her memory.

Even after her mother recovered from the fractures, Valerie didn't see how she could send her mother home. Todd was adamant. "It's her or me. I can't stand always playing second fiddle to an old lady." Valerie could hardly believe him and begged for his help. Instead he left.

Divorce is a frequent consequence of caregiving. Some people just aren't able to allow their homes and spouses to change so radically. Except in the elderly, where death leaves many widowed, divorce rates soar when the need for caregiving is present.

....

How could I decide — my husband or my mother? At first I agonized but then I realized that if he couldn't give of himself to her, he wouldn't give of himself to me.

Responsibility

Many people who need care are not mentally incompetent. What they need is physical assistance with life's everyday activities.

The mentally responsible patient has a new role, too. We should sit down and discuss each person's role. Because personal care is often quite intrusive and degrading, it is better if the recipient gives permission for it.

The patient needs to become knowledgeable about his medical condition so he can report changes either to the caregiver or directly to the physician. This should be the responsibility of the patient for as long as he can handle it.

. . . .

Allowing the care recipient to handle as much responsibility as possible makes my burden easier and the patient can remain an active member of the health care team.

Golden Years

For years we scrimp and save for our retirement. With our expected longevity these days, most of us can anticipate close to two decades more of life after retirement. Pensions, retirement accounts and Keoghs will, we hope, provide funds for our golden years.

But we did not plan for one of us to need continual caregiving. So we become caregivers and watch our carefully thought out retirement funds and fun go down the tubes.

Unless the care recipient is incompetent mentally, there are dozens of ways that caregiver and recipient can travel. Arrangements can be made with a travel agent who plans trips for people with handicaps.

. . . .

While skeptical at first, we decided to try it. With careful advance planning we had the time of our lives. We can still travel!

Hidden Feelings

"We don't need any help. I can do it all. Please leave me alone," Tillie snapped at her daughter Roxanne. Roxanne was always offering to help, to take her father for the weekend, to take them shopping, out to eat or to a movie.

Instead Tillie chose to martyr herself, letting everyone know how hard her new job of caregiving was and staunchly maintaining her ability to do it all alone. Finally their family physician intervened and coaxed her to join a support group for people who are grieving.

"Grieving? I'm not grieving!" she yelled. But at the first group meeting she learned that she was, indeed, going through grief. She was grieving her husband's lost health, their lost retirement years and in this case, even the loss of her lover.

. . . .

No one person can do it all. I know that now and am willing to accept help.

MARCH 7
Another Fall

A recent television commercial shows a situation that some people, unfortunately, have perceived as humorous. It shows a woman who has fallen and can't get up.

In real life this is not funny. Falling is a very real and dangerous problem for the elderly. As one woman dialed the police once again to help her 200 pound husband off the floor, she certainly wasn't laughing. She would have given anything if she could have done it herself and not needed to ask for help.

In her small town everyone knew everyone else and the police always came and gently eased him back to bed. She knew it was only a matter of time before she would have to find alternative arrangements and the knowledge made her feel sick.

....

The saddest day of my life will be when we are separated permanently. While it hurts to know the time is coming, I am working hard to face the future with an open mind.

Reading Aloud

Reading is a wonderful and quiet hobby that many of us enjoy. Even as caregivers, most of us still need to read, although we don't often have the time. We may be chagrined to suddenly find that our loved one can no longer handle a book alone.

Setting a short time aside each day to read aloud, perhaps the morning newspaper or chapter from a book or a new magazine, can still bring great joy.

Reading aloud can give both people a sense of satisfaction and of sharing, once again, one or more mutual interests.

. . . .

Both of us feel more in touch with each other and with the world around us. Current events and good stories make us happy that we can share some of our precious time together.

MARCH 9

What Ifs

At times we all suffer from the What If syndrome. What If I hadn't been at that stoplight just then — maybe the accident wouldn't have occurred. What If I had been injured or even killed, who would take care of my mother then?

It's normal to suffer from a mild case of the What Ifs as we move through our lives, from wondering what would have happened if we had married someone else to minutely examining the details of an accident.

But if we let the What Ifs run our lives, if we spend more time musing than caregiving, we may be caught up in denial of reality. If facing up to caregiving causes too much psychic pain, support groups or a counselor might really help.

....

The only way to face the future is to just face it. Some days are good and some harder but I know I can persevere.

Inventory

Those familiar with 12-Step programs understand the importance of "taking personal inventory" in order to recognize one's shortcomings. Perhaps taking inventory can be defined slightly differently when it comes to caregiving.

For example, if our strong suit is physical care but we dislike cooking and shopping, then admitting that we can't do it all and getting a family member, friend or home health aide to help with those chores is a good solution.

Conversely, if smaller tasks are our forte, or if our own health problems won't allow lifting, perhaps getting that kind of help would balance out the caregiving with our own needs. There is a solution for each problem but sometimes we must look long and hard to find it and put it in place.

. . . .

The positives in my life usually balance the negatives as I find creative ways to care for my loved one and meet my own needs as well.

Shortcomings

The day may come — usually more difficult than most — when I must question my motives and my ability to continue as a full-time caregiver.

When hayfever season came around, one woman who was allergic could barely tend to her own needs. Each autumn she struggled to find some help with caregiving, for had she not, she would have caved in healthwise. Her illness was not within her control. Poor health, mental or physical, demands some sort of assistance.

At such times we might consider moving our loved one to a nursing home, a board-and-care facility or having a student or another person live in to help with the chores.

. . . .

It is really my uniqueness and humanness that make me what I am. I will not chastise myself for what I am unable to do.

The Child Within

Caregiving can sometimes feel like a trap, especially if we are not yet fully realized adults. It doesn't matter how old we are, unless we have dealt with the past's ghosts, we can't be as effective in caregiving as we would wish.

Recognizing old problems and working to heal them, letting our inner child out so that we can acknowledge our past pain, resentment — maybe even abuse — will allow us to give more freely of ourselves to others.

Once we have satisfied the needs of our inner child, whether by journaling, by attending seminars or getting the professional help of a counselor, we can then become more effective as mature and responsible caregivers.

....

Understanding that my inner child was still in pain and needed to be addressed has been a growth and life-enhancing experience. I feel relieved now that I have found the missing piece of my life.

MARCH 13

The Counselor

It is certain that when we are experiencing psychic pain — deep emotional pain — we need help to resolve the problem. We can hardly be effective in a caregiving role if we are barely able to function on our own behalf.

Perhaps it is our anger and frustration about having to be a primary caregiver that has caused the problem or perhaps it has come from expecting too much of ourselves. The fact is, we need to acknowledge it when the emotional pot boils over or is out of steam.

Few of us can heal ourselves or even arrive at an understanding of our problems by ourselves. A real understanding of why we feel as we do can usually only come once we receive professional help.

....

At first I didn't want to see a counselor and thought I could do it all myself. I understand now how crucial it is to feel inner calm and a sense of contentment about who I am and what I need to do.

What creates stress for one person may cause another to thrive. Some people can only function properly when they are on the go, first at work and then all evening and weekend at home. They rarely sit down, let alone relax. Perhaps they don't even know how.

Some might be stressed when the person for whom they are caring has a rough night and they have both been sleep-deprived. Sleep is precious to us all but some function better than others after a sleepless night.

What matters here is not what causes our stress but how we deal with it. If we internalize it, we could be headed for stress-related medical problems or we might be headed for an explosion, like an overhot furnace, and spew venom at our care recipient. Neither does any good. Solving our problem helps.

. . . .

I have learned stress-reducing methods such as biofeedback and relaxation therapy. They have served me well and saved me often.

MARCH 15
Nurturing Ourselves

One important thing that is often overlooked when we are caring for someone else is our own health maintenance. Dealing with our personal needs while our lives are virtually consumed by the needs of another is almost impossible.

If a caregiver has severe arthritis, for example, and does not keep up on range-of-motion and other mild exercises, that individual's health is likely to go downhill, leaving less energy and strength to be a caregiver.

Nurturing ourselves, caring for our health, allowing for a brisk walk, fine music and a good book or lunch out with friends are crucial to staying balanced, even while we caregive.

. . . .

Before anything else I must care for myself or I risk losing my physical and emotional well-being. If that happens, I won't be any good to either of us.

Meeting Needs

There was a time in our lives when we would have laughed if someone else predicted how our days would be spent in the future. Caregiving was the furthest thing from our minds.

Now we can't go to sleep without first thinking through whether we have met all the needs of the person for whom we are caring, so that our chance of getting a decent night's sleep is optimized. Have we put water by the bed? Is the nightlight turned on?

Then, when we do fall into slumber, it is likely we will be called to help, often more than once. Groggily moving through the house, trying to stay awake to give what assistance we can and crawling back into bed again, we wonder whether we will ever get a full night's sleep again.

. . . .

Looking for a solution was the only way to save myself so I found a student to live in and share night duties with me. Now I sleep better and can give better daytime care.

MARCH 17

Temporary Caregiving

Occasionally the need for caregiving is temporary. Perhaps a loved one has broken a hip and is recuperating at home or has had major surgery and needs some special care for a few months.

Most of us are able to rise to the challenge, especially because it has an end in sight. We can be generous with both time and attention since we know that life will soon get back to normal.

Others dealing with long-term chronic illness might need more intense caregiving on and off. As the illness flares up, the need for help is greater. Again, we rise to the occasion, knowing that although the illness will continue, this crisis will end.

....

It hurts me that my loved one suffers from ongoing illness but I am always relieved when the need for intense caregiving is over. With pride, I know I can deal with each new situation that arises.

Handling A Crisis

Although we may not like admitting it, we have settled into a routine of caregiving and have found a way to take some time to fill our own needs. Caregiving is the new pattern — the rhythm — of our lives.

When anything happens to upset our comfortable routine — the care recipient has a heart attack or a serious automobile accident — then handling the situation may be harder than we'd like to think.

Now we are frightened, unsure of what tomorrow will bring, and we become, once again, aware of the fragility of each life. We may pray, we may cry or we may hold all our feelings locked inside.

. . . .

While I would like life to be as it was before, I know that is not possible, so I try as hard as I can to rise to the occasion.

77

Friends

So many caregivers complain that their friends leave them once they become full-time caregivers and the very people they need most are no longer part of their life. Friends are sorely missed — now, more than ever.

This happens for several reasons. Some people, for example, cannot stand to see pain or to watch a good friend's health deteriorate. It may be hard to see a caregiver perform this new job, not knowing how to help.

There are ways to keep some of our old friends. Being honest about feelings helps. Finding time to be alone with friends is another way. Keeping both our interests and our friends is important to well-being.

....

At first I felt isolated and angry at having to caregive and I may have driven friends away. Now I have learned I must take some time for myself and I can spend some of it with a friend.

Frustration

No job on earth can be more rewarding or more frustrating than caregiving. We literally put aside most of our own needs, perhaps even a job we like, to care for someone we love.

Caregiving can be rewarding if the person we are caring for can thank us and participate in the care process. It can be doubly frustrating if, because of the medical situation, that person can no longer relate to us on an adult level or perhaps not at all.

Caring for someone who no longer responds or who has become childlike or violent is one of the hardest forms of caregiving. Few can do this job alone.

. . . .

I felt like a failure when my fatigue was overwhelming and my frustration level high. Getting some help with caregiving saved me and lets me be a better caregiver when it is my turn.

MARCH 21
Cover-Up

Often the individual who is giving care isn't entirely well either. This problem is prevalent among the elderly. Pain and fatigue can be overwhelming and it is easy to rationalize about using medicines.

Just one sleeping pill tonight, we might reason, or some pain medicine, just to help for today. This is human and justifiable, yet all too often our use of medicine becomes more and more frequent and before we know it, we are hooked.

Overusing medicines to cover up anger, pain or fatigue is not a good permanent solution. It can not only be very harmful to the caregiver but the care recipient might also be harmed. A person who takes too much medicine should not be the one giving care.

....

My doctor helped me recognize that I was overusing medicine. She helped me regulate my use and suggested I see a therapist and get some help in the house. I did both and am doing fine.

80

Burnout

Steven had a phone call late one evening from his mother, who was in hysterics. "Steve," she sobbed, "I can't do this anymore. Come over here, quick!" Alarmed, he rushed over.

"What is wrong?" he asked. "Why are you crying?"

Still sobbing, she told him, "Your father doesn't know me any more. He hits me and he hurts me all the time. I just can't do this any more."

Needless to say, the family was stunned and chagrined. She had been hiding the truth in order to "protect" her children, so that their lives were not "ruined" too. The children knew a decision had to be made immediately and recognized that their mother was really at risk — a hard situation to comprehend and deal with.

....

In a nursing home, I can see my husband as often as I wish but I go home alone. It took a crisis for me to see the need.

MARCH 23
Safe Sharing

Some people think caregiving is a "piece of cake." They adapt to the problem easily and move right into the role of being the primary caregiver. For others, however, caregiving is a very difficult emotional experience.

Regardless of whether it is easy or hard, eventually most of us will have some strong feelings and an intense need to talk about it with someone else. The question is — who is it safe to talk to?

We all need to express our feelings and hopefully we have been directed to a caregiving group or even a grief support group. There we will find others who share our feelings, who understand why we are angry or hurt or sad.

....

I feel safe when I share my feelings with other caregivers for I know they will neither judge nor shame me. Knowing I can safely share how I feel lets me be a better caregiver.

Gaining Strength

Besides support groups for caregivers, there are many other places where we can go to get help. There are books available for caregivers, offering both practical advice on how to actually give care and information on how we can care for ourselves.

This may not be enough for some, so we need to remember that our family physician as well as psychologists, social workers and the clergy are available to give spiritual and emotional support.

Admitting that we need help to get through this very trying time of life is not a shortcoming but an individual strength. No one can do it all alone. Each and every one of us needs outside support.

. . . .

At first I was embarrassed by my need for outside support. Now I understand that getting help is good for us both.

MARCH 25

Visualization

Like a fly caught in a spiderweb, caregivers sometimes feel so trapped they can no longer envision any other way of life. On the positive side, those who still have a rewarding relationship with the care recipient can hardly imagine their life without that individual.

This is where visualization, or what our parents used to call daydreaming, comes in. By taking the time to rest, letting our minds wander, we can create any scenario we wish. Visualization can help us come to terms with our life circumstances and can also help us imagine what life might be like if the time comes when we are alone.

By directing our thoughts where we want them to be, time spent visualizing is important and sometimes quite calming.

....

Guilt overwhelmed me at first as I imagined my life without caregiving but soon I understood that visualization is one way for me to escape, even for a few moments, from the tensions of the day.

Improvisation

The topic of sexual relations comes up frequently among caregivers and care recipients. Often the desire is great but the flesh just won't cooperate. This, however, does not necessarily mean the end of a physical relationship.

There are many ways to make love and they need not include intercourse. From pleasuring one another to caressing and holding, couples who are creative can find new and exciting ways to express physical love to each other. There are no limits to the solutions.

There are no rules here other than, "If it hurts or shames either person, don't do it." Otherwise, any way two consenting adults choose to show their caring for one another is quite acceptable and often wonderful!

. . . .

We have had to redefine, for our own use, the term lovemaking. Now that we are learning new ways of satisfying one another, both of us feel more content and gratified.

MARCH 27

Gradual Change

We might not even have recognized or named it yet but when the time comes that another person depends upon us for a good portion of personal care, we have most assuredly become caregivers.

Often the need for caregiving creeps up gradually, just as the symptoms of a progressive disease get worse over the years. First, it might just be help getting up from a seated position and before we know it, we are also giving bathroom help and assistance to bed.

When the need for caregiving comes gradually, there tends to be less resentment than when a person is catapulted into caregiving. But all caregivers and recipients need support — emotional, physical and spiritual.

. . . .

I know my loved one would care for me if the tables were turned. I give care lovingly.

Organizing

Everyone thought she was the strongest and bravest person alive. From the time Helen's husband had a stroke, she was at his side. He could no longer speak but they found their own unique way to communicate.

Friends and family marveled at her ability always to keep a happy smile on her face. What astounded them most was how well she kept records. In fact, her days were over-run with record-keeping. The medicine schedules, doctor's appointments, symptom diary and insurance papers were enough to keep any individual busy.

But her daughter saw through her mother's behavior and told her brother that their mom was using record-keeping as a means of not facing what had really happened to their father. She was right.

. . . .

For months I tried to hide from the truth of our situation. I am beginning to understand that this is our life now. I am beginning to accept the truth.

Guilt

Most of us have heard of survivor guilt, when those who have survived a major incident feel guilty because so many died or when a single family member survives a house fire or plane crash.

What we are less familiar with is the guilt that sometimes comes when one member of a family is sick and the others remain well. The healthy ones may feel guilty for still enjoying good health, for being able to be up and around at will.

Thoughts arise of "Why my loved one? Why not me?" This type of guilt is another unique way we humans have of making our adjustment. It is basically a form of denial and eventually does end.

....

At first, I wondered, "Why us?" Now that time has passed and we have both adjusted, we no longer wonder. "Why not us?"

One More Day

Almost everyone can dig deeply into their personal resources to make it through a crisis. There isn't a mother alive, for example, who doesn't recognize the feeling of weakness after a child has passed a crisis and she can finally let down her guard.

With caregiving it's a bit different, for even as we call on our personal resources, we know that the need for caregiving is going to go on and that it won't be just for one more day.

However, by taking each day as an entity, by breaking down large tasks into smaller, more do-able ones and by not planning too far into the future, we can still operate on a "just for tomorrow" basis.

. . . .

I get frightened if I look too far ahead, so I look at only small sections of time. This helps me to keep up hope and lets me be a stronger caregiver.

Support From Others

"Sometimes I get so bogged down in the minute details of caring for someone else that I forget to take my own medicine!" confessed Howard as he sat in the circle with other caregivers.

Smiling, Chris quietly intoned, "I forget to eat sometimes." Others nodded in agreement.

Molly said, "I remember — but I'm too tired to eat so I just go to bed." Several people nodded in sympathetic understanding.

Caregiving is not easy, yet so many people try to do it all alone, with no outside support. Everyone needs support. After all, when we were in the work force, we had co-workers to commiserate with.

....

I still need my "co-workers" to offer support and sympathy. The members of my support group really help me.

So Alone

Our new role of being caregiver to another person is often confusing and frustrating. Sometimes gradually and sometimes suddenly, we become attached, almost umbilically, to another human being — one who depends totally upon us.

Most caregivers report feeling lonely in their new role, with little or no time anymore for fun, for going out with friends, for eating dinner out or shopping and seeing a movie.

It is this sense of aloneness, of frustration at not being able to live our lives as we please, that causes the most difficulty. Telling our family members how we feel and asking for help and emotional support is a good start.

. . . .

While I feel gratified that I am doing a good job caregiving, I am also tired and lonely. Learning to identify my needs and discovering how to get them met are a good first step.

APRIL 2

Personal Limits

Even before we became caregivers we each had personal limits. These built-in limits indicated how much we could be goaded by our teen-aged children, when we should quit running and start walking. They helped us deal with finances and kept our emotional and physical boundaries healthy and stable.

Our teenagers knew exactly how hard they could push us and they also knew from our tone of voice when to quit. We knew when we had too much sun or when we were too tired to drive. Our personal limits felt familiar to us; they were a part of the rhythm of our lives.

Now that we are caregivers we have to re-learn our personal limits — and when we do, we have to push past them. Giving care to another person is fatiguing and often robs us of desperately needed privacy and sleep.

....

Even though I knew my past limits, I have had to learn new ones. I am struggling to reconcile my needs and my recipient's needs.

Five Million Of Us

One of the most overwhelming things we feel about caregiving is that we are so alone, that no one in the entire world can understand how difficult — though often rewarding — the job of caregiving is. Not surprisingly, most caregivers express the same feelings.

It is estimated that in the United States more than five million people are in the position of giving care to another person, five million families whose lives have been usurped by illness or accident.

Understanding the scope of the problem helps us to appreciate the multitude of support programs and services which have sprung up in the past few years. The need for caregiving will continue to grow and hopefully support services will be developed further.

. . . .

While I try to look at our situation philosophically, I am still the one who gives care. Support services have helped me maintain my sanity and my health.

APRIL 4
Not At Home

It is often assumed that the only people who are really caregivers live in the same home with the care recipient. This is not necessarily the case, since a caregiver might be a neighbor or a friend.

There are many elderly people whose adult children take them shopping — or shop for them — and take them to the doctor. These are the folks who prepare meals several times a week, phone at least once daily, change sheets and do laundry.

Failing health does not necessarily mean going to a nursing home. If the family is willing and has the time, the fortitude and the energy, the care recipient can remain at home, with assistance.

....

We take care of my mother and my father-in-law. It is hard but very gratifying work and we intend to keep on caregiving this way.

A Cup Of Coffee

Most of the world's conflicts, it sometimes seems, could be solved by two mature adults sitting down with a cup of coffee and a strong willingness to compromise. Coffee and a friend provide a unique resting point — one we are familiar with.

In the same vein, many of the caregiver's difficulties seem diminished when time is taken to sit with a good friend or fellow caregiver over a cup of coffee. Secrets can be shared for we know they will go no further. Frustrations can be shared as well.

Not all the problems endured by caregivers need professional intervention or assistance. Sometimes a cup of coffee, a willing ear and a warm hug offer the best help of all.

....

I know I can share all my feelings, openly and honestly, with my best friend. It helps me to know that I have a friend who cares so much about me and about my wellbeing.

APRIL 6

Co-dependency

Without realizing it, some of us are in co-dependent relationships. We may not even have known it, yet for some reason we needed what a co-dependent relationship offered.

By making excuses for a spouse who drinks, covering up for one who uses drugs, turning our heads to real and possible dangerous problems, we demonstrated our tendency to be co-dependent.

If we were already in a co-dependent relationship and the need for caregiving is directly related to illness caused by substance abuse, we may be exceptionally angry both at ourselves and at the person we give care to. We may feel guilty but aren't sure why; we may blame them but aren't sure we are right.

....

If only I had known about co-dependency, maybe I could have been out of our relationship sooner. Now I am trapped but I will still try hard to give good care.

Signals

Most children at about two or three years of age are ready to be toilet trained and parents are alert to the signals a child gives before wetting or having a bowel movement.

Signals are important for all of us and we use them in ways we may not even be aware of. The way we sit on a chair, for example, might indicate how tired we are. Sighing might be a sign of pain, frustration or a way to seek attention.

Like all of us, our care recipient will often signal a need he might not even recognize, from the need for toileting or napping to expressing discomfort or frustration.

. . . .

Learning to read my loved one's signals was hard at first but now the signals help me stay alert to each need. By noticing signals I can be a more effective caregiver.

APRIL 8
Health Changes

Not all health problems are stable. Some, by their very nature, are progressive. In general, we anticipate that a person with health problems who already needs a caregiver may very well get worse.

Sometimes we unknowingly accept changes in health and reprogram our caregiving efforts to fit the recipient's new needs. Over time, the task may become so enormous that we finally realize that one person cannot do it all any longer.

Getting help from a family member or home health aide may be the answer. In other instances, the patient cannot be kept safely at home and it is necessary to consider nursing home placement. We can still continue to give care but we are no longer primary caregiver — the nursing home staff takes over.

. . . .

I can be with my loved one as often as I wish and I can still give care but when I need to, I can go home with no guilt.

Being Aware Of Symptoms

Some people who are incapacitated may have a lessened ability to communicate with their caregiver. This may be the result of a brain atrophy, a stroke or an accident that leaves the individual unable to speak clearly. There may also be impairment in understanding.

Such a situation puts caregivers in a troublesome position, since we must stay alert to any health changes shown by our recipient. Whether it is loss of appetite, fever or something else, it's up to us to identify that there is a problem and call the physician with the details.

When the doctor calls, we may be hard-pressed to describe the problem even though we know something is wrong. Often he will ask us to bring the individual to his office so the problem can be identified and treated.

....

A careful team approach between me and the physician assures that we are working hard together to keep my loved one as well as possible. I appreciate not having to do this alone.

APRIL 10

Criticism

Here is a situation that happens over and over again. Our adult children have just been over to visit and they quietly pull us aside to mention that there are "some things we need to talk about."

With patience and all the maturity that young adults can muster, they criticize our method of giving care. Hurt and now a bit uncertain about how we are giving care or whether we are doing enough, we carefully begin to think over what they told us.

Criticism from people who are not giving care need not always be listened to. Putting what was said out of our minds, we can get on with our task — caregiving the best way we can.

. . . .

No one who is not participating in the caregiving process has a right to tell me what to do. I am doing the best I can.

Fear Of Abandonment

From the day we are born, all humans have a fear of abandonment. As caregivers we have all but abandoned filling our own personal needs. Additionally, we notice that inadvertently over time, we have abandoned our family and close friends.

Becoming a caregiver is not something we ever planned on or expected. Taking care of another person's needs may still feel uncomfortable, even alien, to us and, not surprisingly, we may feel as though that person has abandoned us as well.

The need for caregiving can creep up very insidiously. Before we know it, our entire life seems to revolve around taking care of another person. Many of us pay a high price emotionally.

. . . .

Once I realized what was happening, I worked hard to rectify the problem. With careful work I have slowly drawn family and friends back into my life.

APRIL 12

Unfair Expectations

No one who has not been a caregiver has the right to criticize us, yet all too often our family members expect us to act in certain ways — ways they feel are more correct.

In fact, our family members may not have a good understanding of the toll that the job of caregiving takes on an individual. They expect us to be the way we used to be.

Putting unfair expectations on us only compounds the problem. After all, who has time to bake cookies, make bread and homemade stew and then take little Jimmy to a feature cartoon? Unless the family wants to share in the caregiving, they have no right to expect more of us than we are capable of giving.

....

I cannot be who I used to be or do what I used to do. What you see is what you get. Caregiving is very hard work.

Practical Solutions

It's astounding how much we can learn from others in circumstances similar to our own. That is one reason caregiver support groups are so crucial to our wellbeing.

Going to a caregiver support group may not be simple. Advance arrangements need to be made so we can leave the house. But advance arrangements are worth it so we can hear how others cope with the same problems we have.

From advice on bed-making and bath-giving to strong emotional support for one another, caregivers get back at least as much as they invest in their support group. Support groups offer everything from practical tips to personal lifesaving skills.

. . . .

I didn't realize how lonely and isolated I had become until I joined a caregiver support group. Each time I go, I learn more and feel better about myself and my job of caregiving.

APRIL 14
Tax Time

This may be another first for us — paying income taxes when we are no longer "gainfully" working, due to our need to be a caregiver. We may inadvertently be under-utilizing those funds we do have set aside for emergencies, as well as any savings we may have.

For example, any individual who is medically certified as permanently disabled has a right to withdraw an IRA and other retirement funds with no early penalty. There is a special state and federal form to fill out after obtaining the exemption.

Working closely with an accountant, especially during the first year of caregiving, can be a benefit. A certified accountant at tax time can literally be a financial lifesaver.

....

There are often free tax assistance meetings sponsored through local senior programs and community centers. Tax Help Lines right into state and federal tax offices are thorough and very helpful.

Depression

Fatigue, tedium and even the joy of caregiving can cause a worn out caregiver to lose some aspect of her health. No one can do it all alone but we might not be aware of that fact — yet.

A mild ongoing depression in the caregiver can develop and become a clinical depression. We may not even be aware this is happening since we take for granted the feelings of being run down, fatigued and saddened by our life circumstances.

Clinical depression is a medical problem which can only be helped with medical assistance. No amount of rest or tender loving care are enough. People who are clinically depressed need medical help.

. . . .

For fear that my loved one would not get adequate care, I let my own health problems slide. Now I see that I should have sought medical help long ago. I am now.

APRIL 16

Blame

Some caregivers blame themselves for their loved one's medical problems — I should have taken better care of him and made him eat right — I should have noticed she was run down, that something wasn't right, but I always took her being there for granted. These lamentations do no good for anyone.

No one can force another to eat right or exercise more. Each person is responsible for his own actions, for his decisions on how to live. We shouldn't be willing to shoulder another's blame now that we are caregiving.

Unforseen incidents such as a fall or an automobile accident can happen to any one who is in the wrong place at the wrong time. No child, spouse or parent of that person should carry unnecessary guilt.

. . . .

"I am not now and never was responsible for my loved one's behavior." I used to give that statement lip service. Now I truly believe that I am not to blame.

The Used-To-Be

Now that we are caregivers, there are parts of our lives, our "before" lives, that we may have to give up. This, of course, depends upon how serious the need for caregiving is. With only assistance in some daily activities, our care recipient may be able to manage if we wish to continue working — at least for now.

If, however, the need becomes more intense, it is obvious that we will need to move into a new phase, one in which our role will be that of primary caregiver. This may not be easy but we can certainly see the need for it.

It is normal to mourn the Used-To-Be's of our lives — We used to be such a happy couple — She used to have such a good job — He used to be so self-assured. Having mourned, we can then move on.

. . . .

While I desperately miss good health and my previous lifestyle, I understand the crucial importance of being a primary caregiver and am willing to do it as well as possible.

APRIL 18

Good Sex

Needing another person's help with personal care and everyday activities does not necessarily imply that the warmth and spontaneity of a marriage are gone forever.

As the couple begins to adjust to new norms, they will also adapt to a new lifestyle. Their marriage can stay just as strong as ever provided both can communicate and participate mentally.

Very often a couple — even a couple in which one is a caregiver — can enjoy a good marriage and find creative ways to continue enjoying a mutually satisfying sex life as well, limited only by the physical illness and how imaginative they can be.

....

At first I thought our sex life was over. But we have always been creative and together we have discovered new and interesting ways to fulfill our mutual need for touching and for sex.

Bad, Bad Sex

Chloe didn't know how she would have survived without her Alzheimer's support group. She was relatively quiet the first few times she attended but her fellow caregivers gave her warmth and unqualified love and she quickly learned to trust them.

"All he has on his brain, it seems, is having sex with me. I've been able to brush him off the way one would a child behaving inappropriately. I hated doing it, but any sexual feelings that I have are washed with sadness and with pity for our situation.

"Then," she went on, "one day he rushed me and tried to take me by force. I was badly bruised and very frightened. I screamed. My next-door-neighbor heard and called the police. My husband was temporarily put in a psychiatric unit until better placement became available."

....

The day my very sick and beloved husband used force on me was the day I finally knew we could no longer live together as husband and wife.

APRIL 20

Spring Walks

People who live together for a long time, whether as husband and wife, lovers or parent and child, often develop mutually enjoyable rituals that they look forward to.

Whether holiday traditions, sharing marketing and cooking for special events, gardening or doing inside work together, tradition and habits are an integral part of the tie that binds.

One couple particularly enjoyed gardening and taking long walks around a lake. Now the wife was in a wheelchair as the result of a stroke. Undaunted, they started platform gardening, with her role that of Sidewalk Supervisor and Waterer. The after-effects of her stroke didn't keep them from going walking, either. She rode in her electric cart and they were able to keep their sense of joy and were often seen "walking" around the lake together.

....

Only lack of accessibility keeps us from doing what we want to do and going where we want to go. Undaunted, we just keep on keepin' on.

Vacations

Some families take a long vacation every year, while others plan one only every few years. Some take very long vacations; others enjoy — or can only afford — long weekends.

Vacations can be rejuvenating or they can leave us physically drained and emotionally disappointed. This is true whether we are both physically fit or if one of us is a caregiver and the other a care recipient.

Planning the entire trip ahead — especially if there are special needs that must be considered — can make the vacation better and less exhausting. Expectations that cannot be fulfilled are left out, so there is little disappointment.

....

Realistic expectations and very careful advance planning have allowed us to vacation every now and again. While it's more difficult than before, vacationing can still be wonderful fun.

Double Duty

It happens more often than we imagine. One person is taking care of both a parent and a spouse, or a spouse and a child who also has some special caregiving needs.

Torn between the two, not sure how to split the hours so that everyone gets a share of help, the job is extremely arduous, especially if one of the recipients does not live with the caregiver but instead is miles away.

Not uncommonly, many caregivers in this situation reach a breaking point and can no longer handle the Herculean task they have chosen to perform alone. At the breaking point, they finally ask for help — not a moment too soon.

....

Before I knew it, I was embroiled in caregiving duties. I nearly lost my health; I did lose my sense of wellbeing. I am getting better now that I have asked for help.

Bowling

One of America's all-time favorite pastimes, along with attending baseball and football events, is participating in a weekly bowling league.

With groups of old friends or on a company team, more people than one can imagine look forward to their bowling league night. Giving up the fun of such an important hobby can be devastating, a great loss.

Imagine the joy of being asked to be scorekeeper — perhaps with a bit of assistance — especially when we learn that there are ramps adapted and approved by the American Bowling Association for use in competitive team bowling.

....

Being part of the group and not being ostracized can make all the difference in our daily outlook. Feeling wanted by others helps us both to function better.

APRIL 24

Day Trips

It's almost a crime that so many of us live in large cities and haven't ever taken advantage of all the wonderful cultural, sports and sightseeing activities that are right there.

With a fair amount of safety one can say that most New Yorkers, for example, have never explored all the museums, gone to Ellis Island to see the Statue of Liberty, gone to see the Empire State Building or Rockefeller Center.

Planning day trips in and about our immediate geographical area can be fun and intellectually stimulating. We may need to take one extra person along for emotional support or physical help. Adding more shared new experiences, with a bit of advance planning, enhances our days together.

....

Again, adapting our new life circumstances to other ways of being together and having fun strengthens our relationship.

Group Homes

Sadly, the day may come when it will be clear that we cannot serve as primary caregiver any longer. Perhaps our own health is failing or we may not have the energy or tremendous physical strength required to continue the hard job of caregiving.

Now we are forced to make a decision. It might be best to place our loved one in a nursing home. To many, this is not acceptable, yet, or they may have promised each other — perhaps unrealistically — never to place the other in a nursing home.

At this difficult time, some lucky folks find, in their community or nearby, an approved senior live-in group home. A group home can meet our needs and allow us to honor our mutually given promise.

....

Although still a caregiver, I am not the primary caregiver anymore. This allows me more freedom, yet I can still see my loved one as frequently as I wish.

APRIL 26

New Perspectives

Our daily lives used to hum along with regular routines and patterns. But when the need for caregiving begins, our normal and comfortable patterns, our knowing what to expect on a daily basis disappear and are replaced with confusion and discord.

Many of our life patterns are challenged daily by the overwhelming needs of being primary — often the sole — caregiver. If we are lucky, we can rise to this new challenge without severe damage to our own health, our patience and our personal needs.

Developing new perspectives and perhaps even new goals — perhaps shorter term ones — keeps both of us in better shape. Looking at life with new and different eyes can help as well.

....

Facing each day as it comes lets us both fully experience each day as it presents either joy or sadness.

Hiring Help

There is a very large untapped market for relatively inexpensive assistance and this is the teenage market. Getting a teenager to cover for two to three hours several days a week can be a wonderful way to gain some free time.

While we nap, grocery shop, lollygag in a bubblebath or just do some yard work, teenagers often can fill the bill and be conscientious and very willing workers. And they love earning money!

Playing board games over and over, playing cards or just going for a walk — all three people can benefit greatly from the change of pace, from knowing there will be a break in the day. Having teenagers to help provides relief to everyone.

....

Teenagers can and do bring their fresh and youthful perspective to the job of caregiving. To pay for and receive their boundless enthusiasm and patience is just wonderful.

Slow Going

When we realize that our care recipient is going downhill mentally, suddenly our wonderful everyday rituals — reading for example — seem a burden.

There are ways to handle this problem. The first is to allocate a certain time each day for reading aloud. Reading may be slower but the joy may be greater. A neighbor, friend or a person hired specifically to read for a while each day is one excellent solution.

Another possibility is "Talking Books" — a special home radio service sponsored by state offices for people who are blind, visually impaired or physically handicapped — available free for home use to qualified individuals. From reading the daily newspaper to best sellers, this service is invaluable over time.

....

As I investigate, I am amazed at how many services there are. It's very important for us both to maintain as much independence as possible.

"Guilting" The Recipient

Certainly the last thing we ever intend is to make a person we adore — the very person we are giving care to — feel guilty for being ill. We both know the situation can't be helped.

Yet the person we love, the person we are caring for, is much more susceptible now than ever before to our moods and signals. Without meaning it — the set of our jaw, a word spoken in haste or any unkind movement — may be seen as another reason for the recipient to feel guilty.

Care recipients who are intact emotionally and cognitively but who have physical problems that require help from another person are particularly susceptible to feeling guilty.

....

It simply is not true that I blame my loved one for my having to give care so I need to be certain my loved one knows that.

APRIL 30
....
A Hard Move

After a time, it may become obvious that a two-story house, for example, with conveniences somewhat inaccessible, just won't do now that one family member needs so much help.

One choice is to move into an easier-to-care-for home where necessities are more accessible and conducive to independent living.

Another choice is an intermediate care apartment where one or two meals are served communally and nursing care is generally only a pushbutton away. With planned activities the opportunity to make new friends and supervised outings in special vans and buses, life can once again be new and exciting.

It takes bravery, strength and deep personal commitment to undergo a move which will certainly cause adjustment problems but it is worth it in the end.

....

I pray that my loved one and I will be able to sit down and talk about this before circumstances force us to act.

Prayer

Many caregivers report that prayer or meditation have helped them through the hardest times. Whether caregiving by choice or need, the time spent alone with their God replenishes them.

Reaching the highest possible spiritual plane used to be the defined goal. Now "meditation" has many meanings and is used on many different levels, from occasional deep relaxation to daily meditation, or twice daily, with a personal mantra.

Prayers for strength, for patience, for improved health for oneself or a loved one or for long life are a common thread among people of all religions and cultures.

....

Caregiving is a common denominator everywhere in the world, bringing us together as we share similar problems. Knowing that others are also giving care to their loved ones helps me get through each day.

Spring Gardening

We all grew up hearing that "April showers bring May flowers." April can be a lovely month or a long one, depending upon where we live. If waiting for May flowers is important in our lives, we can start our seedlings right in the house as April begins.

Windowsill planting to get a jump on Mother Nature is a wonderful way to herald spring's imminent arrival. If it is too hard to plant an outside garden, then windowsill gardening can take its place.

Herb gardens are wonderful. Kept on windowsills or some other sunny location, herb gardens offer good payback for very little care. The joy of cooking with freshly chopped herbs adds satisfaction and joy as one more way of adding flavor to our cooking and to our life.

....

Taking a chance on the less-is-more theory, we start herb gardening together. It's a small but wonderful step to keep us connected with nature and with each other.

Potluck

One area in particular that caregivers, and often recipients as well, complain about is a dramatic loss of social contacts. Feeling excluded is a very common problem.

Partly, this happens because we inadvertently let our friends slip away. Our uncertainty in describing what is going on and our lessened physical energy both tend to make us pull away — often without realizing that we have.

Instead, we can be open with our friends and family by telling it like it is — not hiding — and inviting them over to watch TV or play cards or perhaps even inviting them to a potluck dinner. Using paper plates and letting friends bring the main course will keep us involved and let us continue participating in social interaction.

....

It seems we are living a potluck type of life these days. Unsure of what each new day will bring, we can still look forward to entertaining together in a brand new fashion.

MAY 4
Sharing The Day

Overwhelmed with the actual task of caring for another person, we may get so drawn into the caring aspect as to forget our need for the sharing aspect of life.

If our care recipient is able to participate in his own care, he should have a say in every possible decision — What do you want to wear today? What shall we do today? Shop? Go to a movie? Watch that television program you like so much?

By drawing our care recipient into the process we have accomplished two things. First, the recipient is encouraged to share in the decision-making process, even in mundane daily details. Second, both of us are helped by sharing. Continuing to share feelings helps everyone concerned.

. . . .

My care recipient's feelings and needs may be too often overlooked. I try hard to include my loved one both in daily decisions and daily care.

Fear

Calling the police when her gentle and loving husband suddenly became violent, Marilyn was terrified, saddened and repulsed.

Now this irreversibly mentally ill man who had been so important a part of her life for three decades, a wonderful husband and father, was taken away to a locked facility. A head injury in an auto accident two years before had made Carl increasingly violent. As the months passed, he became more distant and frighteningly physical, unlike the man she loved.

Finally she had to admit that her life was in danger. With barely enough time to get herself together emotionally and financially, she'd had virtually no time to grieve the end of their life together. Watching Carl hauled away like an animal in a straight-jacket made her sit down and sob. She didn't know what to do now.

. . . .

Our life as we knew it ended with the car's impact, but the impact upon my life has been great and it will be a long time before I can heal.

MAY 6
Two Disabled Parents

Four years after their mother's stroke, it appeared to their adult children that their parents were adjusting well. She could still help a bit and their father had shown his true colors in taking over the running of the household entirely.

But when their father needed quadruple bypass heart surgery, they suddenly had two parents needing significant caregiving.

As the weeks passed, these grown children developed a deep respect for what both their parents had suffered, first from the stroke and then the heart surgery. The rehabilitation process was difficult and lengthy for both parents and the young folks learned an important lesson in how two people in love can continue to love each other and care so very much.

....

Filled with awe and respect, we realize the superhuman efforts our parents put out to forge a new lifestyle, without imposing on others. Caregiving is not an easy job.

Creatures Of Habit

We are such creatures of habit. Every year a woman lopped off both ends of her Easter ham, seasoned the middle and placed it in her roasting pan to bake. Asked why, she said, "My mother always did it that way." When asked, *her* mother said, "Because my roasting pan was too small, honey!"

Creatures of habit! We buy products we knew as children and are only lately becoming aware of environmental and health issues. Most of us still miss fried chicken, white gravy and homemade mashed potatoes!

Change is never easy but this is a good time to find better ways to be efficient and conserve personal energy. We need not be as fussy about the house, and food preparation can become simpler.

. . . .

*As I continue adjusting to my new role,
I am eager to learn from others in similar
situations. Lowering my expectations and
allowing shortcuts help.*

MAY 8

A Child's Innocence

Older grandchildren may have been lucky enough to know their grandparents as healthy and independent adults but the younger ones or the great-grandchildren may only remember them as ill or debilitated.

It is amazing that children seem able to accept grandparents for whoever they are, for whatever they can or cannot do. And young children pitch right in and help.

From stepping right in, if need be, to feed a grandmother or walk her to the bathroom, even listening to the same stories repeated over and over, the innocence and trust diplayed by children is wonderful. They always manage to find a way to show their love and devotion. The love between a child and a child like adult is a very special sight to see.

....

Any relationship with a grandparent is a bonus for a child. Once illness takes over, the child's overall acceptance incorporates the illness into the whole package.

Autonomy

The feeling of loss of self — losing control over much of who we are and what we can do — can easily take over when a person becomes a caregiver — especially if the need developed suddenly.

For years we strived to make something special of our lives, to achieve our goals, to develop a sense of meaning for ourselves. As caregivers we may have a hard time watching all our carefully laid life plans slide quietly out of our reach.

Maintaining autonomy is crucial now that we are so afraid of losing it. CEOs of large companies, teachers, firefighters, secretaries, maids — we each liked and needed the feeling of pride and importance we felt at work, supporting ourselves and possibly our family.

. . . .

I cannot be as independent as I was, since another person totally depends on me. Slowly but surely I am developing a new sense of autonomy as I understand the importance of being a caregiver.

129

MAY 10
Priorities

An old song tells us, "My how you've changed, my how you've changed." These prophetic words couldn't apply more to the job of caregiving changes virtually every person it touches.

Developing new life priorities is not easy when our underpinnings have been abruptly pulled away. One way we can help ourselves is to work out a brand new scale of priorities.

We may have to give up unreachable goals — such as gourmet cooking or an immaculate house — but we can still feel a sense of personal satisfaction doing our new job well, with warmth and caring.

....

Doing my new job well is my new life priority. As I become a better caregiver, I will try to remember that for every loss, there will be a gain in self-respect.

130

Harmony

We all want harmony in our lives and while we may have had harmonious lives before we became caregivers, life as we knew it then may be gone forever.

For a while, it may have seemed that we would never have a feeling of harmony again. We resist change and continue to struggle with our perceived loss of harmony, autonomy or personal importance.

But eventually, we notice that some of the most gratifying times of life can happen when we give care to someone we love. Slowly a new sense of harmony appears — if we let it — as we are more and more successful in our job as caregiver.

....

Caregiving is a lofty and painful job. Doing it well and graciously allows harmony back into our lives.

MAY 12

Predictability

All in all, most people tend to lean toward a predictable and very safe lifestyle. Choosing predictability over the less stable life that is possible when we must function as caregivers is no longer an option.

A totally predictable life really isn't in the cards for many of us. As soon as we become complacent and settled, our predictable lives change due to the need for caregiving.

Caregiving — the very fact that we have chosen or been pushed into it for lack of any other volunteers — presents many new life options. We have to decide if we are open to change.

....

Caregiving offers a new way of choosing a predictable life, a life that benefits more than one person, a life that can be filled with importance and joy.

Looking For Joy

If we are a caregiver to a loved one, especially if we live together, we will almost certainly live also with a sense of frustration and anger unique only to this job.

We can carry on in this way, allowing frustration, a sense of having lost our right to a real life — a life that included the expectation and even the assumption of wellness rather than illness — to overwhelm us and keep us from doing a good job.

Or we can choose to rise to the top as cream used to rise to the top of an old milk bottle, expecting parts of our lives to remain rich and joyful, expecting satisfaction from a job well done and expecting more happiness than sorrow in our lives.

. . . .

As in other times in my life, my positive attitude is pulling me through. This in no way minimizes the hardship of full-time caregiving but instead gives me the strength I need to carry on.

133

MAY 14
Power Play

Let's face it. Some people are just not happy unless they are in charge — with power over a situation or a person.

Ironically, these are the people who resent it if they have to give up a job but ultimately they enjoy caregiving more than they expected. These are the ones who know that taking full care of another person, taking charge, having control over the care recipient, gives them a strong sense of personal power and strength.

Sadly, in a few cases, these may also be the people who are physically or emotionally abusive or who are so demanding that they actually endanger the health of their care recipient — because of their need for power.

....

At first I had trouble taking care of another person's needs because I was not meeting my own needs. Now I know that to keep my life balanced I need not be so powerful, only loving and understanding.

Vulnerability

At no time in our lives are we as susceptible to stress and fatigue as when we are 24-hour caregivers. When our stress level gets too high we may feel quite emotional and out of sorts.

We may be in failing health ourselves or we may just be tired and overworked and this is the time when we are especially vulnerable. We may at this time have special difficulty making decisions, personal ones and those that affect others as well.

This is the time when we most need help with caregiving. When we are completely worn out, we can't be effective in taking care of another person since the most important rule of caregiving is that we must take care of our own needs first.

Admitting that I am human is okay. I can reach out for help in order to protect my own health and meet my own needs.

MAY 16

Facing The Truth

The scenario is played out in thousands of doctor's offices each and every day. "Your husband (wife) has Alzheimer's disease. We don't know how the illness will act or how soon care will be needed but care will, eventually, be needed full time."

Reeling with the news, husband and wife — or parent and child — try to deny the reality of what they have just been told. In one way, we believe the physician but for a while we choose not to believe, to put off any decision-making, at least for right now.

Finally we understand that the diagnosis is correct and that life as we knew it has changed forever with that single sentence uttered in the doctor's office. It feels like a life sentence and we are overwhelmed with sadness and fear of the unknown.

....

I recognize this illness as truth but denying the diagnosis helped me regain my sense of equilibrium so I could begin making plans for care as time passes.

Decisions

In the beginning when we are just starting out as caregivers, we spend months in virtual isolation, first to get used to the idea of being a primary caregiver and then because we were not sure how to handle this new situation with our friends and family members.

Once we get used to our new role we have many decisions to make. How do we want to conduct our days, for example? With as much normalcy as possible or by hiding our care recipient away in the name of protection?

And who do we really think we are protecting — our care recipient or ourselves — from possible hurt or criticism? It serves no one to become reclusive, for we and our loved one will get on each other's nerves if there is no break in our daily routine.

. . . .

At first it was hard for me to even imagine living a "normal" life again but now I see that life is what you make of it and I am ready to get out among other people again.

MAY 18

Embarrassment

Their son had stopped by to ask if his parents would like to go out to eat with him and his small children. To his surprise, his father yelled, "No! I absolutely do not want to go. Your mother eats like a two-year-old. She embarrasses me in public. If you want to take her, go ahead."

The son did just that. He scooped up his frail, sick mother and off they went for dinner — without Patrick. At first Pat felt guilty; then he realized how much strain he had been under. He was glad she had a chance to go.

Seeing his beloved wife act like a child had opened a wound that Pat could find no way to heal. But those feelings are common. No one can be a perfect caregiver all of the time, thinking only of his care recipient, never himself.

....

We are all vulnerable, especially when caregiving. Showing our human side — our hurt, even disgust — is normal.

Admitting The Truth

Some people get really frazzled just living their everyday lives. Imagine how we caregivers feel, trying to live our lives, with the added burden of caring for another person and filling their needs, too.

Pretending that nothing is wrong, that life is hunky-dory, only perpetuates a lie to ourselves. We can go about and pretend but eventually the truth will catch up with us.

It is now time to stop pretending even to ourselves, that life will ever be as we knew it before.

....

The sooner I admit to myself that I can still function and have an enjoyable life even as a caregiver, the sooner I can get on with living my life.

MAY 20
Self-Pain

Not intending to, but definitely reacting to
how we were raised as children, we bring to our
role of primary caregiver all of our background,
the negative aspects as well as the good.

Virtually the only way we can overcome a
shaky, mistrustful or poorly grounded childhood is to gain understanding of why we act
the way we do and then to learn to own our
current behavior and unlearn some of our childhood training.

This is by no means easy, requiring that we
unravel childhood feelings of not "being
enough," with our intense need to "do it right"
for the person we are caring for. Caregiving
presents a double whammy if that person
happens to be a parent — one who contributed
so much to who we are today.

....

It is hard to heal self-pain but if I am
willing to work at it, I can help myself.

Lack Of Sleep

Plagued by lack of sleep, today's caregivers often become the care recipients of tomorrow. Everyone needs sleep to heal from the rigors of the day. Some need less; some need more. Sleep deprivation will always create problems in the long run.

As we work hard to be the best caregiver we can be, we also tend to give up more personal rights than just the right to a good night's sleep. Privacy, sometimes even in the bathroom, is often one of the first rights we miss, followed by lack of time to spend alone, just reading or listening to good music.

There are creative solutions to this problem: hiring someone to stay overnight, permanently or every now and again, so we can get some rest or placing our care recipient in a respite care facility for a few days.

....

Feeling restored can mean everything and a few nights of uninterrupted sleep can bring new calm, patience and endurance to my role as caregiver.

141

MAY 22

No Guilt

The thought of taking a vacation without our soulmate, our confidante and support, may feel like blasphemy. How can we even think of such a thing?

Reason prevails after a while, however, as we think of how much more effective we could be if only we were rested or had more patience. So we think of how it would feel if we did, indeed, take some time away alone.

On the other hand, if we choose to go away with our loved one, we can make the best of it and enjoy a good, quiet vacation, even if only for a few days. We will come back refreshed.

....

I never thought I could admit that I feel refreshed and renewed by being away from the stress of life at home. It is good for me to get away for a while every now and then.

Commitment

To the question, "Will you love, honor and cherish one another until death do you part?" we answered "I do," but what if we do not stay healthy until death? What then?

It is not always death that separates a couple. It can be the disability of one partner and full-time caregiving required of the other. And caregiving was not in our marriage contract.

Given no choice when the crisis occurs, we may think once again about our marriage vows. Some people do, unfortunately, choose to leave as soon as a health problem or injury arises. Others, more deeply committed, recall the importance of their marriage vows, of sharing both the good and the bad of life and they stay.

. . . .

The love and devotion I feel from caregiving come from a deep commitment to going through life together — caregiving or not. I am proud that I care enough to stay and help.

Bootstraps

Some people feel so safe, so lucky, that they can transcend any life situation, including the need to caregive. When asked how they manage to stay so seemingly happy, these indomitable folks often respond, "Well, I pulled myself up by my bootstraps and stepped right in and did what needed doing."

Impervious to the needs of anyone but our care recipient, we jump right in, expecting that others will share our optimism and do what is right — jump in and share the job with us.

We may be surprised to find that not everyone feels as we do, not all people are capable of being caregivers. Those who can't should not be belittled for each of us can only do our best under the circumstances.

. . . .

I always want to do my best and prove myself capable of doing the job yet I remain pleasantly surprised at how my sense of caring and my sense of commitment have become one.

Rewriting Marriage

Unlike the man who leaned over his wife's casket lamenting, "I should have told her how much I loved her, how much she meant to me," we needn't wait until death for our final goodbyes.

Caregiving offers an excellent way to demonstrate our feelings to a person we love very much. Our caregiving, our patience — even our voice — can provide a way to rewrite our roles in marriage as a caregiver and care recipient.

The need for care may last for years, perhaps even decades. What a marvelous opportunity to right old wrongs and begin again on a new footing.

. . . .

Only I can decide how I will treat my loved one both in and outside of my caregiving role. I will be as patient and loving as possible.

MAY 26
One In Twenty

Morning again. Stan wondered how he could get up and face yet another 24 hours of caregiving? He lurched into his morning routine, wanting to cry, not at all sure he could handle one more day.

Caregiving can be terribly hard, even when we enjoy caring for the person and that individual is responsive and participates in the care. Stan knew he had to see their family doctor and tell him what was going on.

In the company of millions — in fact, one out of 20 people — Stan was suffering from clinical depression which was heightened by his need to be the fully responsible party in his marriage. Getting some counseling, taking prescription medicine and having some time off each week gave Stan a new outlook on life.

....

I was mistaken to think that the way I felt was due to being a full-time caregiver. Now I know that I must listen to my body and get help when it signals me that something is wrong.

What About Me?

It was a complete reversal of situations. Her husband of 40 years, whom she had loved and cherished through bad and good times, had become her caregiver. Diabetes, blindness and an amputation had made her an invalid.

She lamented to her children, "What about me? He goes about cleaning as if I were a piece of furniture. He won't listen to me. What about what I want?"

Wisely, her children suggested they all sit down for a family council. Their father joined them and listened to what they had to say. "Honey," their mother said, "I'm disabled, not dead. I can still think and I can still contribute to the running of our home. You are making me feel unneeded — like a fifth wheel."

. . . .

I am embarrassed that I took over so completely — but I was only doing my best to help. From now on I will consider my wife's needs too and we will work out a plan together.

147

Care Plan

The disabled sometimes feel burdensome to their caregivers and this may, in fact, be true. When someone who was active and successful needs help — often even with the most personal needs — it is demoralizing and debilitating to them.

Now caregiver and care recipient, and often the physician as well, need to sit down and form a plan to encompass everyone's needs. First, of course, is safety and medical care for the disabled person, but the life-care plan should also include recreation, outings and sharing laughter.

Caregivers need to be reminded that laughter is important. Humor and fun should not be unimportant. Balance is the best plan of all so that each one's needs are met and each feels valuable and worthwhile.

....

Our life can be happy and well-rounded,
even when there is a need for caregiving.

Don't Say That!

"It would be better if I died. Then you wouldn't have to worry about me. You'd live a good life without draining your savings," cried the grown and very ill daughter of her parents, her primary caregivers.

"Don't ever say that!" they both barked at once. "You did not bring this illness on yourself and while we wish we could take it from you, this is how our lives are right now. We couldn't imagine our lives without you, so be quiet and help us make the best of a hard situation."

Their daughter sobbed with relief. When the crisis set in, she and her children had moved back to her parent's home. She needed almost full-time care and both parents shared in care-giving. She was so relieved to know how much she was still loved, even if she never got better.

....

Taking care of an adult child who is very ill is a sorrow for everybody concerned but if we remember to talk about it openly and express our love for one another, we will do fine.

MAY 30

Journaling

Many caregivers are emotionally bottled up and may need an outlet for feelings. Journaling can provide it. It costs nothing, one can do it whenever there is a spare moment and it is a wonderful way to chronicle our successes, our failures, anything we want to write about. Care recipients can journal, too.

One disabled woman started writing poetry in her journal. Years after she died, her children found it and it was precious to them for it showed a side of their mother they had never known.

There are classes to help people get started in journal writing. The thoughts we put in a journal are not meant to be shared, although we certainly may share them if we wish to.

. . . .

My journal has become my confidante, a place where I can express my secret thoughts without fear of being censored.

A Caregiving Mentor

A mentor is someone who has special skills or unique experience who is willing to help us as we begin our journey.

Some people are mentored through reading a book, others as new parents. We may find someone who has been a caregiver and will help us get used to our new job and seek the right resources.

Anyone who has tried to contact the right social service agency to ask a question or obtain a service knows how frustrating this can be. Along with helping us learn about caregiving, our mentor has probably made all the calls before us and can provide information.

....

Surprisingly, my mentor was someone I barely knew, yet he had heard of my plight from someone else and was kind enough to offer his help. I never could have got such a good start without him.

JUNE 1
Responsibility

In our society women are far more likely than men to become long-term caregivers even when they need or want to work outside the home. Millions of women are in this position these days.

Many working women use most or all of their salary to pay for help or a daycare program for a husband or elderly parent so that they can have health insurance and bring home a salary. Still, that is a very arduous path amounting to two full-time jobs.

Predictably, the eventual price for these women is their own failing health and inability to keep their jobs. There is little comfort in knowing that so many millions share the same predicament.

....

I can only do the best I can. By continuing to work I can hold on a bit longer to my sense of self-worth but when the time comes to stop, I will do so with no regrets.

Attitude Readjustment

How many times have we heard, "Just hold on and be grateful. It could be worse. I know someone who . . ." This is not the kind of talk we need to hear as we struggle along trying to make the best of each difficult day as a caregiver. We need sympathy and understanding right now, not stories about other people.

Others don't realize that we don't need an attitude readjustment. What we need is an offer of real help, of time with our care recipient so we can get out. Instead of criticizing, they should try walking in our shoes for a few hours.

Even though people want to help, to cheer us up, what they unknowingly do is make us feel bad that our loved one needs so much care and we are the only ones available to give it.

. . . .

Gratitude doesn't come easily when I am so fatigued but just for today I will try to find something to be grateful for. It might help.

JUNE 3

Don't Tell

When friends ask casually, "How are you doing?" we might accidentally answer them with the truth. We know it's only a casual question, not expected to be answered truthfully but sometimes we are sorely tempted to tell them.

It takes time and perspective as a caregiver to learn what our new role really is. We are learning to behave differently, both toward the person we are caring for and toward those who ask facile questions. We fear that if we break down and tell them how hard it really is, our friends will leave us.

So we keep our own counsel and only confide in those few who are very close, those who are in and out of our homes, our hearts and our lives. To them, we owe the truth.

. . . .

I will keep my own counsel when people need not know all the details of caregiving but I will tell when it matters to my well-being or the well-being of my loved one.

154

Future Loss

Caregiving involves a mourning process. We mourn for all we have lost, the hoped-for future good times together, the lost financial security, the loss of our future and the loss of our loved one as he or she used to be.

But caregiving need not be only loss. Many people find that it brings great joy to help someone they love. Some report feeling closer than ever during the caregiving period.

However we see caregiving, it certainly can be a time of rampant emotions, from the highest highs to the lowest lows. It helps to learn to move through what each day has to offer without worrying too much about tomorrow.

. . . .

What I make of my caregiving experience is up to me. I have the right to feel all my feelings and deal with them any way I wish.

JUNE 5

Will It Happen To Me?

Everything affects everything else in life. When we are in the position of being a caregiver for someone who used to be a completely capable, autonomous individual, we wonder, for one thing, if it will ever happen to us — if we will need a caregiver.

Change is inevitable in life but when the change includes caregiving, the sheer number of changes may seem almost too much to handle. The more difficult the changes our lifestyles undergo, the more likely we are to develop a stress-induced illness.

Each day we work hard to accomplish all our tasks and be certain that our care recipient is well cared for and safe. Each day we pray that it will get no worse, that things might — just might — improve. If they don't, our physical health is likely to suffer eventually.

....

I know that I am overtired all the time. I promise to listen to my body's signals and take good care of myself.

156

Losing Our Niche

As caregivers, we may, quietly and without realizing it, slide away from our old life, our old friends, from all the things that used to be important to us. We don't mean for this to happen but our days are overtaxed with all the work of caregiving.

Many people pull away from all their other roles, from being a parent, from being a job holder, even from going to church or synagogue. This is not intentional — there just are not enough hours in the day nor enough people to help.

It hurts us so much that someone we love dearly is in such trouble. We almost feel it as our own pain — in fact, in a way it is. Caregiving is hard.

. . . .

I know it is important not to lose myself in my caregiving role. I will find someone to relieve me so I can have a few hours off each week.

JUNE 7
Support

It is so important to have support from others — family members, friends, perhaps paid professionals.

It helps immensely to have people around and especially when they understand that we have needs, too. Recognition for the good job we are doing and practical help are both essential.

One of our most vital needs is for company — for friends and family to come and be with us, even as we caregive, even to bring along a meal or stay to play cards or watch television with us. We don't want them to take over, only to share some of the trials and agonies of our caregiving job.

....

Having those who love me come around from time-to-time regardless of how ill or inappropriate my care recipient is, lets me know that I am loved.

Crisis

Crisis happens. Sometimes even a minor problem can escalate into a real crisis and when it does, we need to have a plan of action ready.

We need to know from the family's physician what constitutes a medical crisis. Knowing when we should call for help gives us confidence. The crisis might even be our own, not the patient's. We may become ill or fall. We may be "out of it" emotionally for a while.

Having a plan makes things easier. A little rain might suddenly become a full-fledged storm and we need to be certain our flashlights and rowboats are in place before the rain begins.

....

I used to be an excellent crisis manager but now that I am always so worn out, I have set up a plan with our family physician and with family members that can be put into motion in moments.

Barriers

Caregiving support groups are essential for many of us. These groups offer several things. One is the company of others who are in similar or nearly identical situations and understand what we are going through. There is the promise of new friends who really understand what we are going through.

In these groups, there are also trained facilitators who can offer practical help for common problems.

There are some obstacles which keep people from getting to a support group. They might not have anyone to fill in at home or a way to get to and from the meeting. But caregiving support groups are very helpful and if a way can be found to get there, we will be happy we did.

....

I had all sorts of excuses for not going to a support group until a friend offered to pick me up. Now I couldn't make it without my support group friends.

Where To Turn

For every problem in life there is a solution but sometimes it takes about a hundred phone calls to find help or the answer that we desperately need!

There is nothing more frustrating for an overworked caregiver than having to spend half the day on Hold, only then to find that we've been connected with the wrong department. We have so little time to spare.

There are social service agencies who have some of the answers we need. Senior advocacy groups might be another place to look for help. It takes time and perseverance but we can get assistance or information if we stick to the telephone.

. . . .

My time is so precious these days. I am at first angry that I have waited so long, then grateful that I have finally reached the right social service or senior agency who can help.

161

JUNE 11
The Long Haul

When we start on the caregiving road, we have no idea how long it will be, unless, of course, the situation is obviously temporary — a broken bone, recovery from surgery.

But we are committed for the long haul. If we are having a hard time with that, it is better not to speculate on the length of time but instead to accept each day as it comes.

If we persist in keeping some semblance of a personal and social life, if we get our own needs met, whether through professional help or a daycare program for our loved one, we will be able to be loving and patient.

....

I felt so selfish at first when I sent my loved one to daycare three afternoons a week, but to my surprise, he loves to go and I enjoy my personal freedom on those days.

Sources Of Information

Before our loved one became ill most of us probably had little knowledge of their particular illness. We may have had a general point of reference, how a person with Parkinson's disease walks or the kind of behavior that goes with early brain atrophy disease, but we lacked real information. We didn't have a good grasp of the disease process or what would happen to our loved one.

The organizations that concern themselves with various diseases are remarkably helpful. They send extensive information about the illness, providing seminars, support groups and often phone support — they are available to help when we need them.

. . . .

When I first went to an information meeting, I was a stranger, both to the illness and to the group. They held out their hands to me. Now I have new friends who share problems and solutions just like mine.

163

JUNE 13
Letting Ourselves Ask

Common sense dictates that we can't give or accept help until we are ready. We may start out with a sense of near omnipotence. After all, I love the person I am caring for. Who can do it better than I?

This feeling wears thin after a few weeks or months with little or no sleep, a diminishing social life and rare time to spend alone. Finally we agree that we are, indeed, ready to accept some help.

Whether it's information, practical advice on caregiving or actual physical help from another person, we know that it's time to ask. We may be surprised at what we get when we ask.

....

By letting myself ask, all I am admitting is that I, too, am human.

More Than Competence

When we clean our home we may think that no one can do it as well. When we wash our car, only we know the best way to do it. No one else could do it as well. But as caregivers we may need to give up our perfectionist standards and allow others to offer help.

Sometimes it isn't the level of skill that the helper brings to the job but their compassion, their gentleness, their caring. Even untrained hired people have a tremendous amount to offer, from helping us with tasks to offering the patience we sometimes are too drained to give.

A person who cares about our loved one and comes to love them too is worth her weight in gold for that person often has infinite patience and is kind beyond words.

. . . .

It embarrassed me that I needed someone to help me with caregiving. Now I can't imagine how I would effectively caregive without my assistant.

Loneliness

Feeling lonely is hard enough to deal with but when the loneliness is caused by the fact that as caregivers we have isolated ourselves, it seems twice as hard to take.

We didn't mean to become reclusive — sometimes we are just too tired to make the effort or perhaps our loved one's behavior is so inappropriate that it embarrasses us in front of others.

Loneliness is associated with disturbed sleeping and eating patterns, feeling too sad to function except in the caregiving role. Loneliness can quickly become depression if we don't turn our lives around and give ourselves some time off from this very difficult job.

....

I felt so isolated until I finally forced myself to arrange for two half days of respite each week. I go to a caregivers' support group and I keep time open for seeing friends. I am happier now.

Uncertainty

The sheer uncertainty of our days — and our nights as well — makes us frightened of the future and perhaps even of the present. Caregiving is consuming and each day can be different.

One of the hardest parts of caregiving is that we seem to lose control of our own lives. There is little pattern to our lives anymore except to answer the needs of our loved one.

Life seems uncertain and, in fact, it is. Not knowing how long we will be caregiving or what will happen next week or the week after makes caregiving an especially difficult job to handle.

....

Making some sort of short-term plan and finding a way to implement it, whether we have planned to read a book or take a walk, helps us feel that we are in control of at least part of our days.

JUNE 17
Compromise

When we were young, we didn't much like to compromise. Most of us wanted what we wanted when we wanted it. If we married or began to work with others, we quickly learned the art of compromise, for one can't be with another person without sharing thoughts, feelings, time and often the bed covers as well!

How flexible each individual is predicts how happy or unhappy that person will be in the caregiving role. People who are very easygoing, who can let problems roll off their backs are likely to be able to caregive more easily.

Those who won't or can't compromise, who need to run a tight ship, tend to have a harder time. Many caregivers eventually become master copers, however, since they have little choice.

....

I can't believe how much easier it is now for me than when it was new. Not only do I know how to do it well, but I have learned to let go of my old habits and caregive in new ways.

168

So Sad

How can we know if we are really depressed, and not just sad about our loved one's poor health and our having to caregive? Sadness goes away in a day or two. When we are just sad, a good cry, or sometimes a good laugh helps create a mood change.

When the sadness doesn't go away, when we feel helpless and lethargic most of the time, it is likely that we are depressed. People who are depressed often have a hard time taking care of themselves, let alone another person.

Perhaps we have suicidal thoughts and all we can think about is the negative — or difficult — part of our lives. At this time, we owe it to ourselves to see our family doctor for help. Depression is treatable. No one should have to feel that there is no reason to live.

. . . .

My brain seemed stuck in molasses when I was depressed. Only three or four weeks after I saw the doctor and was given medication, my life improved dramatically. I am sorry I waited.

169

JUNE 19

Just A Nip

It doesn't take long for someone who turns to alcohol when they are unhappy to become a *bona fide* alcoholic. Sadly some people who were forced into caregiving because there was no one else to do it may turn to the bottle for relief from emotional and perhaps physical pain.

It seems so innocent at first, just a little nip. Some people are able to have only an occasional drink and do not become addicted. The problem arises, however, when the bottle becomes our "permanent" temporary solution for dealing with our problems and hiding from our feelings.

A caregiver who drinks too much not only places the disabled person in danger but themselves as well, for their judgment and reflexes will be suppressed. An alcoholic simply cannot caregive effectively or safely.

. . . .

I confess to reaching for the bottle in the beginning of my caregiving job but a good friend took me aside and told me how it looked and how dumb it was. I'm so glad I listened.

False Alarm

What happens when the person for whom we are caregiving says they feel suicidal? What should we, as their caregiver, do about the threat?

All suicide talk should be taken seriously and we should call for help. The physician should be notified for our loved one may need to be placed in a psychiatric facility for a short time. Then we need to sit down with the doctor, evaluate the situation and develop a plan.

Is our care recipient physically capable of taking his life? Does he have the strength, the means and the mental capacity? Or is the word suicide used to get a reaction from us and some extra attention? This is an extremely hard call to make and we can't be on guard 24 hours a day.

....

I was so frightened when my loved one talked about suicide but after careful observation and evaluation by the doctor, we both feel it was a cry for more attention. I am still scared.

171

JUNE 21

Medication

We know how easily a child can be poisoned or even die from taking medicine found lying around or in a purse.

People who are mentally incompetent may be childlike and also take medicine without telling anyone, thinking it is candy, or just because they are too confused to know any better. So we must hide the medicine or lock it up, to prevent poisoning.

How sad the day when we finally realize that our loved one can hurt himself due to childish or irresponsible behavior, through no fault of his. Leaving a stove burner on or starting a fire with a cigarette are other dangers. We need to keep a watchful eye.

....

The saddest day of my life came when my loved one no longer recognized me and was no longer capable of making adult decisions. I am working to accept this change but it is very hard.

Long Distance Responsibility

It is not uncommon for a family, and particularly a woman, to work, take care of her own family and also caregive long-distance for an elderly ill parent. For a time it works, at least until the disabled person can no longer safely live alone. Then it gets extra hard.

There are many options, from hiring another person to live-in as companion, to placement in a nursing or board-and-care home. Even then we are still responsible and the calls and visits become not only expensive but quite draining emotionally.

We must take care of our parent's legal affairs and talk often with the person who is living in or the nursing home staff. The financial and emotional drain mounts. Being caught in the middle is terribly difficult.

....

I wish my elderly parent lived nearer to my home so I didn't have to spend so many hours traveling. But I love my parent and will continue to do my best.

JUNE 23

Confidence

Our confidence may wane temporarily when we begin our new role as caregiver. After all, this job means taking care of another person's life and we don't know how to do it. Such tasks as toileting may be difficult but we soon get used to them all.

Our confidence will grow, however, when we understand and accept the changes that have happened both in our lives and in the health of the one we love. Soon we will feel pride in doing a hard job well.

Unfortunately many of us are not ready to accept the changes as fast as they are happening. Health and needs can change in a flash and it's awfully hard to admit the changes are permanent and our loved one's health will only deteriorate.

....

Only with total acceptance of our new lifestyle can I allow myself to flow with each change and accept it as gracefully as possible.

Peer Counseling

Only in the past ten years have services for caregivers improved. Often there are daycare programs in each community and other support services to help the caregiver.

Among the most successful are the peer counseling programs now proliferating all across the country. Peers are trained to be friends to caregivers as well as active listeners and perhaps problem solvers, too.

Peer counselors come to the home once or twice a month, sometimes more often. The emotional support offered by the peer counseling groups is so great it can hardly be measured. For some caregivers, the peer couselors are their only visitors — ever.

. . . .

My peer counselor is wonderful and has become my friend. Thank goodness for the unselfish people who are willing to give their time.

JUNE 25
An Excuse

It may be surprising to hear that some care-givers give more care than is needed and actually smother the care recipient with too much attention. They rarely leave their loved one's side.

In fact it is not uncommon for a caregiver to use the role of caregiving as an excuse to become reclusive, to avoid being involved with anything but the day-to-day life of being a caregiver.

Talking it over with our loved one might be a very enlightening experience for we might learn that we don't need to give care 24 hours a day. There may be certain things the person cannot do alone anymore but we may be smothering with too much well-meaning care.

. . . .

It took a real reversal of thought to let my care recipient be alone. I am glad we talked and that my loved one can still reason and take responsibility for some personal care.

Adaptive Changes

As we continue in our role of caregiver we might need to assess our house or apartment for safety. Can our loved one go to the bathroom alone? Could they, if there were an elevated seat and grab bars? Are the stairs safe and would a light and an extra rail help?

Any adaptive changes we can make that will allow our loved one to be safer or to do some tasks alone should be made. A high stool to sit on when preparing food, a microwave, grab bars, raising chairs and sofas a few inches — each change that will keep the person independent and safe should be implemented.

Imagine our surprise when the changes are made and our loved one does much better than before! Simple changes, mostly inexpensive, can make a difference to the person who needs help.

....

I was thrilled when I realized how much more my mother could do for herself when we adapted the house to suit her illness. Now we both feel good about it and we both enjoy our privacy.

JUNE 27
The Doctor

The time may come when we spend more time at the doctor's office than ever before. Sometimes it is hard to keep in mind that while the doctor cares about us and our care recipient, he or she is not a personal friend and should not be treated as such.

This is difficult because the doctor will come to know all the details of our daily lives. By not placing unfair expectations on the doctor, by not expecting the doctor to be a mindreader, we can maintain a professional relationship that will benefit us all.

Honesty is essential with the doctor, for hiding feelings or problems helps no one. We should never be tempted to ask the doctor to examine us if the appointment was for our loved one. There is not enough time to examine two people in a single visit.

....

It is hard to get everything ready to take my loved one to the doctor but we are a team keeping my loved one as well as possible.

Medical Goals

If we don't talk to our care recipient about a medical visit and carefully explain what the doctor has said, if they did not understand, we are doing our loved one a great disservice.

Even if we know they can't really understand what we are saying, it is not fair to expect them to grasp what went on without a simplified explanation. After all, they are the reason for the visit.

Getting to the doctor can be difficult what with arranging transportation and getting everything ready. Remembering to include our loved one in the actual preparation really helps keep our goals and the doctor's goal firmly in mind.

．．．．．．．．．．．．．．．

I wish we could have bigger and better goals rather than just holding on to the status quo. Each time I visit the doctor I wonder if the news will be bad and am so relieved when it is not.

JUNE 29

Death

One of the saddest things is when a husband or wife unselfishly devotes years of caregiving to a spouse they adore, yet after a time the disease takes its toll and the person dies, sometimes quite unexpectedly.

When our loved one is gone, there may be a terrific void in our lives. Not all people think caregiving is a chore. They do it willingly and without anger or shortness of temper. Now the one we loved so dearly is gone and we feel lonely.

Beginning to build a new life is hard. Many need to start all over, for their old friends have either moved away or died. It feels as if we're in a time warp for years.

....

Starting over is hard but the same determination I brought to caregiving, I can bring to creating a new life for myself.

Reasons

There are so many different reasons why people choose to become caregivers. Most would think that it is a job they were forced to take by default, that there was no one else to do the job.

While this may be true, the three main reasons that people choose to be caregivers are that they see it as an obligation to a beloved family member, that it made them feel very good to be doing something so important for another person and that by caring for a loved one they may themselves deserve care if they need it.

Each person gets something different from caregiving and each person brings to the job the sum total of all their life's experiences. Some are better at the job than others but most people work hard and do their best.

....

Caregiving was the hardest job I ever had but it also was by far the most fulfilling.

JULY 1
Before The Crisis

The daily newspapers are filled with stories about family members trying to get permission to "pull the plug" in order to end their loved one's suffering or some who are fighting to keep the life supports going even though there is little or no chance of recovery.

Discussing one's personal wishes about these matters is never comfortable but it would save family members terrible grief if only people would do so while they are still capable of expressing their wishes. Life support? Organ donation? What type of funeral? These are hard things to talk about, perhaps, but the time may come when we will be grateful that we did.

While our loved one is still healthy enough to understand and express personal desires is the time when we should each be asking the other these hard questions.

....

I know my loved one is getting worse and I feel reassured that we discussed how we both want the end of our lives to be managed.

Time Alone

The number of caregivers who never get any time off from their task is vast. Many report that it has been more than a year since they have had a few hours or a day just to call their own.

Discussing your needs with your care recipient is often helpful, if the individual can still discuss the matter. Then set about finding someone to come in and take your place temporarily. Try volunteers from among church groups, neighbors and friends and, of course, family members.

It's important that we reassure our loved one that he or she will be well taken care of and that we will be back within a specific time. Leave and try to have a good time.

. . . .

I was frightened when I trusted my loved one to someone else's care but since that first time it has become easier. My time alone is precious and it refuels me to continue caregiving.

Make It Easier

There are services for caregivers that might make the job easier. For example, it would be wise and reassuring to know that we have an emergency system in place so we can push a button for help.

Meals On Wheels is available in many areas and often both people can qualify for it. This way one meal less needs to be prepared each day. Peer counselors often will come in to offer support, friendship and advice.

A telephone answering machine avoids the need to rush to the telephone if we are otherwise occupied. Many places now offer respite care services, both for emergencies and to provide days off for the caregiver. These should help make caregiving easier.

....

It seemed like cheating when I first got Meals On Wheels. Now I see it and similar services as a godsend. They all help make my job a bit easier.

Independence Day

For many of us Independence Day is just another day to caregive. That is fine but there is an alternative. While it will never be the same as when our loved one was healthy, we can still plan to attend a celebration or have a small one right in our own home. Many older people, especially those who are not well, and their caregivers would relish the thought of spending a pleasant potluck dinner with friends.

Even though our lifestyle has changed, we can still have celebrations and stay involved with other people. It may take considerable effort and much advance planning but the rewards are well worth it.

....

The Fourth of July! For the first time in years I am looking forward to a holiday!

JULY 5
Laughter Medicine

It may seem as though there is just no reason to laugh. Our loved one — husband, wife, parent, sister or brother — is ill and we have taken over the role of caregiver. Laugh about what?

When we don't use our sense of humor we lose our sense of joy and hope. Laughter is easy. Making an effort to laugh may sound foolish but that old Abbott and Costello "Who's on first?" routine can make anyone laugh. Bring humorous books into the house and rent video comedies. Read the funnies together.

A few minutes of laughter is a wonderful catharsis in a world that seems more and more confined by the restraints and needs of caregiving. Don't be afraid to laugh. It makes most people feel better, at least for a short while.

....

To my surprise, my loved one laughed with me when we watched a funny movie, even though she rarely expresses any emotions anymore. It made us both feel good.

The Expert

So often roles are reversed when there is a need for caregiving. We may be mowing the lawn one moment and draining a urine bag the next. The chores of a caregiver are many and varied.

By default we have also become the family financial expert even if we never kept the family books before.

We have also become expert at gauging whether something is wrong with our loved one and how serious it might be.

We observe his behavior and call the physician if need be to report anything that is different physically or emotionally. This is not an expertise we ever wished for, but it's probably one of the most important things we will ever do as a caregiver.

. . . .

Jack of All Trades is not a label I ever wanted but I have earned my Expert's badge and am proud of it.

JULY 7
....
Companionship

Even though we are perfectly willing to be a caregiver, for a time our primary task may be just to be there, to be a companion in our loved one's time of need. She may need someone to play cards with or to share a cup of tea with.

"Companion" is a gentler term than "caregiver" and it signifies a different type of watchful caring. A companion shares life, shares living space and shares problems. Caregiving may not be necessary yet.

Not until the person we live with becomes more seriously ill or begins to deteriorate do we actually move up a notch and begin to serve officially as a caregiver. Sometimes the need happens so gradually that we are caregiving before we know it.

....

I don't mind being a caregiver because it happened slowly over a period of years. It seemed easier on both of us that way.

Other Services

Programs such as foster care for adults can help long or short term. The disabled individual moves into the care provider's home and is given meals, close supervision and assistance with personal grooming.

Telephone reassurance programs are now being run in many areas of the country. This is especially worthwhile if the caregiver is also not well as contact is made by phone once each day. Also, there are mail carrier alert services, where a flag is turned over each day by the occupant so the mail carrier knows everything is all right.

Chore services have sprung up everywhere; usually pre-teens and teenagers work for a small fee and do snow shoveling, yard work and other chores that the caregiver may not have the time or physical energy to perform.

. . . .

There are many services available to help me. All I need do is pick up the phone and ask for help.

Family Conference

When the need for caregiving is new to a family, especially if it comes abruptly, it is helpful for the entire family to sit down and talk over their roles.

People can do a better job if they understand the problem, what is causing it and what to expect. Going together to the doctor before the patient comes home will help each family member understand what to expect.

Setting clear-cut tasks for each family member according to ability and setting up goals as well is most helpful. If a teenager knows that her job is helping Mom take a bath and starting dinner three times a week, then she will be more willing to do her share. If the oldest son is responsible for setting and clearing the table and driving Mom to the doctor, he too, will help. Naturally an adult has to be the primary responsible caregiver.

....

My family has rallied and together we will make an excellent cohesive caregiving team.

Chief Caregiver

In spite of the support we get from family, friends and neighbors, we are still the primary caregivers, the ones who are there all the time. In each caregiving case there always needs to be only one decision maker.

There is a fine line, however, between making a decision and being dictatorial. We need to ask ourselves: Am I doing it this way because it's convenient to me or to my loved one? Have I taken my care recipient's needs into account as I plan the day? Do I keep my mood so nothing I do is tinged with personal anger?

If we honestly answer these and other questions, it will be apparent that we might do some things for our own convenience. While our loved one might enjoy a bath in the evening, for example, we need to explain that it has to be in the morning because we no longer have the energy to give a bath at night.

....

Caregiving is give-and-take. I will try to weigh my needs equally with those of my loved one and strike what balance I can.

JULY 11

Special Implications

Giving care to a child or parent certainly can be difficult but often not nearly as difficult as giving care to one's husband or wife.

If it is our spouse we are taking care of, the emotional implications are stronger. This is a person with whom we have shared our entire adult life, whom we have laughed and cried with, reached for impossible dreams with and often accepted less, raised children with and made love with. This is our beloved.

It hurts so much when a person who has been a part of us does not function in that manner any more. This is especially true if he no longer can respond to us as adults. It is one of the hardest things ever to let go of who they were before and accept them for what they can do and who they are today.

. . . .

My sense of wellbeing diminished in the beginning, for I missed our old life so much. After time, I found other people who listen to me and support me if I am going through hard times.

Spirituality

All too often people think spirituality and religion are the same, just as many think sexuality and sex are the same. Sexuality reflects how we feel about ourselves in total whereas spirituality is about how we react and connect to the world around us.

Sometimes, caught up in the rigors of being a primary caregiver, we tend to be too narrow, dealing only with the task at hand. Our sense of spirituality suffers as we pay little attention to the world around us.

Once we are more comfortable with caregiving, we can reconnect with the world outside and marvel at the first crocus of spring, the first robin and the sounds of birds. Just listening to a cricket chirping on a summer night can be a lovely way to connect with the world and experience spirituality.

. . . .

While I was too busy at first to care, I soon began to notice the world around me and I am once more awed at the beauty of it all.

193

JULY 13
A Parade Of Friends

Just as we never were prepared to be a caregiver, we also never were prepared for the parade of strangers who might begin passing through our home in order to help with care.

All the people who come to help, the home health aide, if we can get one, the visiting nurse, if we need one, the physical therapist, the person from chore services, all do their best to make our lives a bit easier. Friends and family might offer to help as well.

They were strangers at first but it didn't take long to realize that together we all are a team — a team that has been custom-designed to make the job easier and to give our loved one the very best care possible. Strangers no more — instead a parade of friends.

....

I marvel at the good work done by the people who come to our home to help. They have helped form the framework for fine care.

194

A Family Condition

When one person in a family has a chronic health problem, especially if their need for care is increasing, the entire family shares the problem. Each family member will be affected in some way.

It won't do to pretend that everything is still fine, for it is not. It won't do to ignore the need for help, for it won't go away. One family member's chronic medical condition is the family's problem as well.

The ripple effect of the need for caregiving in a family will spread to all who enter our home. People tend to pitch in and help without much question. The need is great and the family needs to share the load so the burden isn't just on the primary caregiver.

. . . .

We say our whole family had a stroke, for it did affect each and every one of us. Our love and cohesiveness as a family unit will help us to handle this problem as well as possible.

Living With It

When we receive a diagnosis of ongoing chronic illness, we eventually recognize that we have no choice in the matter, that we must learn to live with it. We don't like it very much but we know there is no choice.

If the illness progresses to the point where we need to have a caregiver, then someone else will be in charge of helping us do some of the things we can no longer do for ourselves, such as personal care or cooking and shopping.

Giving up part of our pride hurts more than just our self-esteem. Losing personal independence is not easy but it helps everyone involved if we can be gracious and thankful for the help we are receiving.

. . . .

Neither one of us likes the illness and what it has done but we are both working hard to continue enjoying a good life together despite the ravages of illness.

Forging The Way

Not unlike the pioneers who opened up the old West, we who are giving care along with our care recipient are forging new ways to work together. This is a do-able task.

By showing the utmost respect for one another, by always considering the other person's feelings, we can demonstrate that we are not there to take over the other individual's life but to share in their problems as well as their successes.

Success is a good watchword for caregivers, since in working together as a unit to provide good care, both caregiver and recipient can feel successful — the care recipient because he can still do some things for himself, and the caregiver in being able to help a beloved person.

. . . .

Looking at caregiving as a way to enhance a relationship, as a way to show love and respect for one another, makes us both feel better.

197

Assessing Needs

Caregiving, much like life in general, is not static. Each day the individual's needs may shift and we have to be ready to recognize their new need and be able to respond fully to it.

When health is the issue, especially if the illness is progressive, we may soon discover that the needs our care recipient had last week are different than the present ones. In general, the trend is to need more care unless our care recipient is recovering from some temporary medical condition.

By assessing our loved one's needs on a continuum, we assure both ourselves and our patient that his care will be consistent and adequate.

. . . .

Just as life changes, my loved one's needs will change. Hopefully I will be able to continue to see the need and meet the challenge.

Stress

When a person we love has a chronic ongoing medical problem, the stress on us is enormous, especially if that individual no longer functions mentally or intellectually as they used to. Watching a person we love go downhill is devastating.

Dealing with the stress of the situation, apart from dealing with their need for us to become primary caregivers, is excruciating. It is often helpful to go outside our home for some help in dealing with such difficult situations.

From chronic illness support groups to those for caregivers and those experiencing grief, support groups are invaluable. We certainly experience grief when a person we have loved is changing before our eyes. We grieve all that was and all that could have been. Support groups offer support in a way no one else can.

....

I never thought support groups were for me until I went to one. Now I look forward to it and expect to leave feeling better.

JULY 19

A Good Attitude

The story is told about the woman who had a serious chronic illness but somehow still managed to be always friendly, have a pleasant smile on her face and keep a positive attitude.

A man whose wife had recently suffered a serious stroke and was now home called on this woman for advice. "How do you keep such a good attitude?" he asked. "My wife is such a grump."

"What kind of personality did she have before her stroke?" she inquired of the chagrined husband.

"She was a grump then, too," he replied.

"Good attitude and happiness come from within," she explained. "Some people are blessed and others not. Don't expect her to change just because she had a stroke. You're asking for the impossible."

. . . .

It looks as though any changing that is to be done in our family will have to be on my part. I will work hard on developing a pleasant and helpful attitude.

Gratitude

The family was in an uproar. The children lived at least five hundred miles away from their mother. Naturally, they rushed to her side after the accident that left her in need of care for the rest of her life.

None of the children had much money and they didn't know what to do about caring for their mother. She could speak and was a pleasure to be with but obviously would need full care. They didn't want her in a nursing home.

Then their mother's best friend stepped forward. "I could care for her," she told them. "I'm having money problems. If I could live with her free and be paid a small salary, it would be wonderful for both of us. I used to be a nurse and I know I can do the job." The grateful family quickly made the arrangements so this wonderful, kind friend could move in.

. . . .

We never know if and when we will be rescued from a dilemma. Bless the friend who was willing to be our mother's primary caregiver.

New Skills

Many people accept that life as they knew it is over. But instead of developing new skills and a new lifestyle, they spend the rest of their lives mourning what used to be.

For one thing, the care recipient might need to have outpatient therapy on a regular basis. Caregivers are generally responsible for carrying out the regime of daily exercise as set up by the physical therapist and this takes some effort on their part.

Even though life will be different, it can still be good. By attending daily to the exercise program, our loved one has the best chance for recovery, and by keeping an upbeat attitude, a new lifestyle can be forged together.

....

It's a difficult adjustment, getting used to living with a person who needs care, but together we are working to make the very best of it.

Choices

Life is full of choices, from the time we are born until the day we die. While some people choose to be a primary caregiver willingly, others simply do it because they have to. So the two people now launch into a whole different lifestyle than they knew before.

Now it's up to them. There are still many options available. Both caregiver and recipient can make decisions about how they want to live their lives. Will you be reclusive? Are you willing to get out into the community, take classes together, go to the movies or concerts?

Life is really what we make of it. Unless the patient is immobile and cannot even go out in a wheelchair, or unless he is mentally incapable, there is a wonderful world out there and all we have to do is participate in it.

. . . .

Once we got used to our new lifestyle and the changes it has brought, we decided to get on with life. It's harder to do so than before, but now we get out and enjoy ourselves often.

JULY 23
Confusion

One of the worst things to be faced by both caregiver and care recipient is when our loved one becomes confused. Confusion may be mild or it can be so severe that it really is arduous getting through each day.

People who suffer memory loss, lessened ability to reason and the ability to relate to others are often harder to care for, especially if they are combative as well. This is an especially frustrating and confusing situation.

In some cases, a decision is made that the individual will not be kept at home, that she needs more care than one person at home can give. In these cases, a nursing home is most often the answer. We still function as the caregiver but not the primary caregiver.

. . . .

I was so confused about what to do but finally I realized it was not even safe for my loved one to stay at home. I had not wanted it to be nursing home care but I really saw no other way.

The Environment

Once we accept that our loved one has deteriorated and needs full-time care — and it does sometimes creep up on us because we are with them every day — it is time to adapt our living quarters to accommodate their needs and ability.

When we think of accommodation, we usually think of grab bars and railings, but this is not always the case. While these things may be needed, we also need to look at the accessibility of tableware, where food is kept in the refrigerator and on the pantry shelves, the height of tables and chairs as well as convenience in getting in and out of bed.

Making a home accessible does not always imply handicapped accessibility but finding ways to keep our loved one as independent as possible by arranging the home to suit special needs.

. . . .

As I went through our home I tried to look at it through the eyes of my loved one. I was surprised at how many simple changes I could make to help with daily living.

Understanding

It is so very important that the caregiver understand thoroughly and completely what has happened and what might happen in the future.

By being emotionally prepared and by finding the best ways to cope physically, we can help ourselves to help them. A hundred pound woman may not be able to lift her two hundred fifty pound husband, so she asks about a hoist that will do it for her.

Looking realistically at our own strengths and weaknesses will help us give the best care possible and also show us that sometimes our best intentions are just not enough. At this time we may need to consider getting help in the house or finding alternative ways to suit our loved one's needs.

. . . .

I wanted so badly to remain the primary caregiver but my physical limitations would not allow it. I have hired someone to help and I can still participate in the caregiving process.

Advance Grieving

While terribly sad, it is true. Some of our loved ones have progressive diseases such as cancer, heart or lung disease and will die in the next few months or years. This is a hard situation.

As we give care, we can't help but notice that our care recipient is losing weight and losing strength as well. We know the end will come in a matter of months. Talking together about the inevitable helps, as does getting one's affairs in order.

Advance grieving, which is what many people do during the time period immediately before death when we know for certain that death will occur, helps many caregivers prepare for the inevitable. This gives time to say goodbye and to begin adjustment.

. . . .

Knowing my care recipient is going to die just tears me up inside but I realize that finally there will be peace for my loved one, who has suffered so much in these past years.

False Pride

It is so hard at first to admit how bad things really are in the house. Our adult children might confront us with what they see as truth but we are not yet ready to admit that what they see is all true.

"It's really not all that bad," we protest. "I can manage without any help." It isn't that we don't know, deep down inside, but we are having a hard time recognizing that these changes are permanent and things are likely to get worse. It is a very sad time.

Protecting our adult children and friends from the truth doesn't work for very long, for if they spend any time with us they will see how quickly their loved one has become worse. Eventually, we must admit the truth to ourselves and make plans to move on.

. . . .

Admitting that my loved one has slipped so far was hard for me to do. The slide from a vibrant useful human being to one so childlike has been very hard for me to handle emotionally.

208

"Let Me In"

It's no wonder our closest friends and family members get angry with us. At first we are so protective of our feelings and of how our loved one behaves. But they know what is happening.

We try so hard to do it all alone, until finally a grown child or dear friend implores us, "Let me into your life. Please let me help. This person means a great deal to me, too, and you can't do it all alone. Let the people who love him help you."

To such a plea we can hardly say no, and suddenly we feel so relieved that their offer of help was forthcoming. Finally we can admit, even if it's just to ourselves, how very, very tired we have become, how sad and scared we are and how out of sorts we have been feeling for lack of sleep.

....

Thank goodness for dear friends who wouldn't let me do this alone. I didn't realize how I had isolated myself in my need to be a good caregiver.

Loneliness

It's easy to delude ourselves, to pretend that eventually everything will get back to normal, to the way things used to be. But eventually we have to admit the truth to ourselves: that life as we knew it has changed forever.

While we are struggling to give the best care possible, we are also having an internal struggle to cope with the sudden loneliness we feel. Our loved one is no longer acting as a spouse but instead has become a person we hardly recognize.

Loneliness pervades all the parts of our life. We can either accept it and continue to caregive without regard for our own personal feelings, or we can take some time off to be sure we are surrounded, at least occasionally, by people who care about us.

. . . .

The loss of my loved one as she used to be was awful. I had to get used to caring for someone I didn't know, someone whose health had changed drastically. It has taken time but I am doing better.

Reality

Our intentions may be excellent but no matter how hard we try, we cannot change the personality of the person we have loved so much, especially if this is a disease that causes brain loss.

Brain loss is so hard to cope with, especially if the individual no longer recognizes us. To have spent a lifetime with a spouse, or to have had a parent upon whom we could always depend, deteriorate in such a way is devastating.

Nothing in life prepared us for caregiving to someone who is essentially a complete stranger. Their body may be the same but their personality is gone forever. It's such a hard, sad situation.

. . . .

The hardest thing I have ever done in my life was watch my loved one deteriorate mentally. I did the best job I could. No one can ask for more.

JULY 31
Roles We Play

We all play a variety of roles in life, starting as someone's child and grandchild, then as student and perhaps soon as boy or girlfriend. Next we often fill the role of best friend, lover, aunt or uncle and then finally, most of us become parents ourselves.

One role change we never anticipated is that of becoming a caregiver, or if we did, we planned on caregiving for our own small children, just until they became independent adults. Never once did we expect to care for an adult who needs our help, especially not for a husband, a wife, a parent we love so very much.

Getting used to our new role is not easy, especially if the individual we are caring for has undergone major physical or mental changes. Caregiving is definitely hard work.

....

Working hard to accept my new role, I am trying to move on.

I Wish

When we confront our shortcomings, we can hardly avoid making statements like, "I should be more gentle with my loved one — I am too short-tempered — I should be more patient but it's hard to do this job alone."

It doesn't do any good to punish ourselves with "I should" or "I wish" statements. For all our wishing that our loved one will improve cannot come true if the illness is progressive. What we want and what reality offers are two different things.

We have to face the truth. Admitting that, at least for now, we are caregivers for someone we love, that things are not likely to change in the near future and that our care is needed will help us face the inevitability and sometimes even the boredom of our job.

. . . .

It seeems like heresy to admit that I hate being a caregiver and that I wish things could be the way they used to be. I am working to make an adjustment but it is not easy.

AUGUST 2
Neglecting Ourselves

When someone we love and who is sick moves into our home, there are major adjustments to deal with. Even if the individual were well, it would be hard having another person living with us especially if we are cramped for room.

Now that our loved one needs us to give care, we usually do so at first with a vengeance, sometimes neglecting our own family and our own personal needs. This need not be the case.

A family council should be held, with each member of the family taking on a new responsibility so that the burden isn't all on one person. We might also hire someone or get a relative or neighbor to give us at least two afternoons a week off, so we can attend to our own needs.

. . . .

Having a loved one live with us is doable providing everyone cooperates and no one feels neglected.

Shame

Most caregivers feel guilty that they may not be doing enough for their care recipient. Regardless of how many hours we spend in actual care, we still feel as though it is not enough — that we could do more.

Shame also enters the picture, especially if our loved one has a degenerative or brain atrophy disease that makes us feel embarrassed to take him out in public. Then, naturally, we shame ourselves because we feel ashamed.

We have to accept the present reality and go about our lives, still going to restaurants, movies and friends' homes, not stay home and become reclusive.

. . . .

I am ashamed of my feelings of shame and am working hard to accept this "new" person into my everyday life.

AUGUST 4

Role Reversal

Most of us like having a mother or a father always there for us. It is a shock when we finally — or suddenly — realize that we essentially now have to switch roles and be the parent, since our parent has become childish and is now the child. This, of course, can be true for spouses as well.

It is hard to be responsible for taking personal care, at least in the beginning, of the very person we have depended on to always be there for us. Sometimes we wish our parent or spouse had died instead, for we are not sure how to handle this difficult new role.

There are no quick fixes or easy solutions. Day by day we make our adjustment until we finally accept that the person we knew and depended on is gone forever. And so we do our job.

....

I miss my mother (or father) so much. I never dreamed I would be taking care of my parents but I am proud that I am doing my job well.

Emotional Support

There is probably no single group of individuals who deserve emotional support more and who get less of it than caregivers do. As caregivers, we give all of ourselves, until our reserves are drained completely.

The habit of asking for and getting emotional support comes hard but help is available if only we will ask. From family members to caregivers support groups to social workers or psychologists, emotional support is abundant and underused.

Like everything else in life, to receive support we must first be willing to admit that we need it and then we must seek it out. We will never be sorry that we asked for emotional support. It will help in countless ways we can't even measure.

. . . .

I really thought I needed no one, that I could do it all alone. I was wrong and I am so happy that I sought emotional support.

AUGUST 6
Mental Illness

Millions of people in the United States suffer from mental illness. The problem is hardest for those who deal with people who are incapable of making decisions for themselves.

Many mentally ill people do improve with help from a physician, a psychiatrist and perhaps hospitalization if they are suicidal or dangerous. Yet when some of these people come home, they may not be able to function normally and it may become our job to care for them. Rather than caregiving, we may feel like watchdogs.

Afraid they might commit suicide, we try to watch them all the time. This is so wearing and bad for all concerned. At this time it might be wise to find alternative living arrangements for our loved one who is mentally ill.

. . . .

Nothing I could do would make my loved one's mental illness go away. When I had to give up trying to help and hoping for a cure, I felt both pained and freed.

Regrets

The feeling of regret that lingers when our loved one becomes chronically ill, is injured or develops a terminal illness is hard to describe. We mourn for all that could have been.

By allowing our care recipient to do what she is capable of doing for as long as possible and intervening only when necessary for safety or personal hygiene, we are showing our respect and caring.

It is indeed unfortunate when a healthy, vibrant person is struck down with a severe health problem and we are so sorry both for them and for ourselves. Regret and sadness at our situation and theirs dominate our lives at this time.

. . . .

When other people commiserate with me, I appreciate their caring but it doesn't change the fact that my loved one has a progressive disease.

Relaxation

When we get so tense that we just don't know what to do, it is a good time to learn about relaxation therapy. Those people who have never read about relaxation therapy or learned how to sit down and go into a state of relaxation just don't know what they are missing.

It is surprising how relaxed we can get just by reading about how to relax and then following the simple directions. It only takes 10 minutes or so of time but is a miniature mental vacation.

The feeling of well-being and of regaining control that we get by giving ourselves this gift daily — even more than once a day — is almost immeasurable.

. . . .

I vow to learn relaxation therapy and give myself the gift of time.

Hope means different things to each of us at different times in our lives. There is a story about a woman who was in so much pain before surgery that she hoped and really thought that she would surely die. After surgery her pain was even greater and she was sorry for a few days that she hadn't died! Slowly she improved and the pain disappeared.

We feel somewhat like this during the course of our loved one's illness. First we hope and pray they will improve or even recover.

Soon we hope they will become unaware of how ill they really are so they won't be humiliated by their own behavior or overwhelmed by their pain. Eventually the hope is for death — quiet, quick and not painful, just that it be over.

. . . .

I can always hope for the best but the "best" changes as my loved one's health changes.

AUGUST 10
New Priorities

It's amazing what a chronic illness of one member can do to a family. Some people pull away, unable to handle the physical or emotional changes going on. Others use illness as a way to create more togetherness.

Many people report that they have never felt so close, so much a part of a single cause, as they have since the need for caregiving arose.

Using illness as a reason to be closer than ever is just fine, so long as the care recipient isn't smothered by our love. Finding pleasures in life's simple things comes more frequently now, as does finding pleasure in just being with each other.

....

I never dreamed that caregiving would give me the opportunity to be closer than ever to the one I love.

Between The Lines

Caregiving offers a unique opportunity to observe and act on certain things about our partner that we might not have noticed before. We quickly pick up and act on signals which might previously have been ignored.

We need to learn to read between the lines of our loved one's communication and actions. Are we filling his needs? Is there any other way we can do a chore that is less uncomfortable for him? Care recipients often do not complain because they feel they have lost that right.

By reading between the lines, so to speak, we can be alert to our loved one's needs. And we should not forget to listen to our own signals, to fill our personal needs as well. We both matter very much in a caregiving situation.

....

I thought I knew my spouse very well until I really began to observe her. I was chagrined to find that she had unmet needs, which I am now working hard to fill.

AUGUST 12
The Gift Of Yourself

How sad that as caregivers most of us don't give ourselves enough credit for all that we are doing. Most of us do give ourselves credit freely for doing the actual tasks related to caregiving but too few of us give ourselves credit for everything else.

We are giving, generously and with love, the gift of our time — time we might have chosen to spend in a different way had we not become caregivers. Also we are giving the gift of caring and of unquestioning friendship.

The gift of touch, of holding, of loving, comes easily, yet we don't give ourselves credit for these, nor for our friendship and hours and hours of our time.

....

I can step aside for a moment and look at all the gifts I have given without thought to my loved one. I feel very proud.

We Can Hope

Whether we are in a caregiving role or not, it is upsetting to see the health of a person we love get worse. All we can do, besides providing care, is to offer our hope that things will get better.

Sometimes there is a reprieve. Illness goes into remission or the person heals from an accident they were not expected to heal from at all. Then, at least for a time, we can offer support but we don't have to hope for a miracle that has already occurred.

When there is no improvement, however, we begin to hope all over again — that our loved one will not suffer too much — that they will feel little or no pain — that the end will be easy.

. . . .

Hope always springs eternal but there comes a time when we hope the end will come swiftly and without too much pain.

AUGUST 14
Touching

Sometimes we are so involved in the tasks of caregiving that we forget about other kinds of touch. Everyone needs to be touched. This is a gift we can offer our loved one.

Brushing a woman's hair or massaging sore shoulders offer touch that is rarely given now that the person is sick. Stroking an arm or a cheek, or if the situation allows, even making love to our spouse, are all ways of touching that we may have forgotten about because our situation has changed so radically.

Touch is such a special gift and one we neglect, both for ourselves and our loved one, now that illness or injury has entered our lives. Remembering to touch brings special feelings of closeness that we may not have had for a long while.

....

I had forgotten amidst all the caregiving work, how important it is to touch. I like touching and being touched and I feel happy that we are becoming close once again.

Losing one's sense of dignity often feels like surrendering totally to ill health and to what has happened. Each person, regardless of how weak they are, regardless of how they function intellectually or emotionally, deserves to be treated with dignity.

It's easy to lose sight of that fact, especially when, as caregivers, we are fatigued beyond words and feeling short-tempered at having to clean up yet another broken glass or change yet another bed.

Being treated with dignity is a basic human right, yet it is far too easy to lose sight of that fact, especially when we are giving care. Perhaps we ought to sit down a while and ask ourselves if we are really treating our loved one the way we would want to be treated.

. . . .

When I finally thought over the issue of dignity, I felt ashamed for I have been guilty of rushing my loved one as one would a recalcitrant child. This will not happen again.

AUGUST 16
Crying

When a person cries and cries, we wonder if that person is in a depression. This is not necessarily the case. Tears are sometimes necessary to help us adjust to something that feels like an impossible situation.

Is the woman depressed who cries often because her husband is dying of cancer? Or is she just normally saddened at the loss she is going to feel?

When a man cries often as he watches his now childlike wife who no longer recognizes him — is he depressed — or is he just undergoing the normal unlocking of pent-up tension?

Tears are normal and healthy when our loved one is very ill. They help prepare us for what is coming. They help us grieve for what we have already lost. We need to cry in order to heal.

....

Crying lets me handle my grief. I am not weak nor am I depressed. My tears are self-affirming and I need to cry.

I Used To Be

There is almost nothing sadder than seeing a loved one go downhill. Remembering that just a few months ago this person had skills that are now gone forever is so heartbreaking.

"I used to be able to do that," they may comment. "I used to be useful." Saddest of all — "I used to be your mother (or your husband or wife)." The individual has no concept that he is still who he used to be, although now in a completely different role.

Hard though it may be, sometimes it is also a blessing that the person's memory is failing for it would be even more tragic if they understood how things are now.

. . . .

What used to be is gone forever. From now on we need to deal with this day and what we can do to make our loved one as comfortable as possible.

Laughing Together

It is odd how many caregivers report that their relative, who rarely showed any sign of having a sense of humor in the past, has suddenly become a riot to live with. Now that inhibitions have been stolen away by illness, humor is found in many daily situations.

Laughter, which used to be rare from this individual, is heard all over the house. He laughs at anything the least bit humorous. It is easier for us to share laughter instead of tears.

What a difference a bit of laughter can make in the attitudes of both the caregiver and care recipient. Laughter shared is laughter remembered.

....

What a gift we received when laughter once again entered our lives. We make it a point to watch funny movies and cartoons together for now we both enjoy a good laugh.

Too Much Tension

It is apparent to anyone who enters the home. The tension is so thick one could cut it with a knife. Visitors no longer feel comfortable so they begin to stay away.

As caregivers, there may come a time when we have to admit, even to ourselves, that we just can't do the job anymore. Our health is suffering even as we watch over the health of our loved one.

Finally, we know a decision needs to be made. Asking family members, or friends if there is no family, and the patient's physician for an opinion, it appears unanimous that it is time for our loved one to go into a nursing home. We hate doing it but there seems to be no other way.

. . . .

I am breaking a promise that I would never put my wife in a nursing home but if she knew how bad her health is and how difficult it is for me to care for her, I know she would understand.

AUGUST 20
Be Happy

"Be happy," they tell us, those well-meaning folks who really do care about our welfare. "It could be worse. At least this individual can walk. What if they had to use a wheelchair? So be happy."

How angry we feel when they feed us such ridiculous platitudes. "Be happy!" Let them walk in our shoes for a few days and nights and find out what it is really like to be a full-time caregiver. We try to hide our anger and be pleasant but it is no easy thing.

Caregiving can be overwhelming or it can be merely another task we incorporate into our day. It all depends upon the health of our loved one. If we choose to be happy it will be because something good has happened to cause our happiness.

. . . .

People are so well-meaning as they remind me to smile and be happy. I try to be pleasant but they really do not understand my anger and how I feel.

232

Anniversaries

For some lucky people, anniversaries can still be celebrated. For although one partner needs to be a caregiver, the other person is fully aware and participates in the marriage in many ways.

Celebrating birthdays, wedding anniversaries, even the anniversary of a loved one's death can be shared, and the burden is easier to bear. There can still be joy or sorrow as we remember together the good and bad times of our life together.

However, when our loved one can no longer participate with us or interact as an adult would, we have to carry the burden alone. Try as we might to ignore the anniversary or birthday, we are still conscious of it all day. Anniversaries can hurt.

. . . .

Try as I might, I cannot ignore the anniversary of the day we became engaged, the day we married and the days of our parents' deaths. I know now it is all right for me to feel alone, lonely and sad.

Pushing

We all know someone who never would have got out of their home, never participated in senior citizen classes or taken day trips, if some friend hadn't pushed them into it.

The same holds true when we are caregivers. Of course, we have to judge when to push and when not to. Perhaps we are pushing for an out-of-the-home adult daycare program and we have to work hard to persuade our loved one to try it just one time.

To their surprise, they love it. Most people, even those who are very ill or losing their mental capabilities, appreciate interacting with other people. We never imagined that it might be boring to just be with us all day, but it was.

....

When we see our loved one's reaction to being busy, how eager he is to go to his program each day, we know we were pushing him in the right direction. It feels good to be right.

Imagine

When we were children, we had such vivid imaginations. A sand hill with a few sticks and some small rocks were all we needed to keep busy for an entire afternoon. Our imagination was rampant with the possibilities for play.

As adults, too many of us lose our capacity for play. Now more than ever, it is important to give ourselves the gift of just letting our mind wander for a while. Let it go wherever it wants, from imagining how life would be if we were not caregivers, if we could still be at work, to going off on an uncharted vacation on a raft.

Let's try to recapture our capacity for play. Try going for a walk with our loved one — a nice slow walk, paying attention to all the beauty that surrounds us. Imagination. What a wonderful thing!

....

Giving myself brief times "away" from my duties as a caregiver is refreshing and important for it refuels me and lets me get to the work at hand.

AUGUST 24

Information, Please

Just when we think we have a handle on everything, just when we think we finally understand our loved one's illness, a new problem occurs which causes us to call the physician or a knowledgeable organization.

Asking for more information shows that we are interested and caring people. What we need to know may not necessarily make us a better caregiver but it will at least allow us to know what to expect.

Those of us who ask for information frequently may find we need more than just information. In this case a support group for caregivers or for loved ones of people who have a specific illness might be in order. However we get our information, it is important to ask if we feel the need.

....

At first I felt foolish asking for information or help. Now I understand that most people need help during the caregiving process and I know that I am not alone.

Religious Fervor

One of the first things to be put off when our loved one becomes ill or injured is attendance at church or synagogue. There just aren't enough hours in the day, we reason, and besides, if there is a just God, how could He let illness happen to a wonderful person?

Before too long, however, many people do a complete turnaround and become more religious than ever before. Every spare moment is spent praying — even silently — that the loved one will get better, will be saved or will not have too much pain. We may even pray that we will no longer have to be their caregiver.

We may lose our need to worship or overuse it because we are confused and saddened that the illness will run its course regardless of what we do and how much we pray.

. . . .

Recognizing the inevitable result of the illness and perhaps the end of life is one of the saddest things ever. There is nothing I can do to change my loved one's health and I feel so sad and frightened.

237

AUGUST 26
Not Telling

"Let's not tell Mom how sick she is," the father said to his adult children. "It will just make her more depressed to know that she is dying." Although they did not approve, the children and the physician went along with his viewpoint for they knew that handling her dying would be hard enough on him.

"Let's not tell Daddy how sick I am," whispered the mother to her children. "I'm not sure he knows the truth. It will be too hard for him to handle the fact that my illness is terminal."

Instead of being able to comfort each other in their time of extreme need, both people were deprived of sharing, caring and the talking over of memories. How sad that the secret was kept to the end.

. . . .

Although my intentions were honorable, not talking about dying when death was imminent did us both a disservice.

Expectations

We can hardly forget our parents' disappointment when they expected us to behave in a certain way and we did not. We knew they had certain expectations but still we misbehaved.

This same thing can happen when two people are married and one becomes ill and needs a caregiver. The sick person may expect us to do something in a certain way and be disappointed when we don't, even though there was virtually no discussion about it. The same is true for the caregiver who might expect his loved one to behave differently than she does or is perhaps even capable of behaving.

Expectations are fine if both people know what is expected and agree to it. It is unfair to expect someone to read our minds or our signals.

....

In order to anticipate a certain behavior, I need to remember that we both need to talk about it and decide together what to expect.

AUGUST 28
Guilty Feelings

It's almost humorous how many people joke about the guilt they feel and say, not without some truth, "I was raised with guilt on the brain!" This is not really the least bit funny yet feeling guilty when our loved one becomes ill somehow is an accepted thing.

It is generally no one's fault when a chronic illness occurs. There are exceptions, of course, as when a smoker gets cancer or emphysema — then we do have the right to feel angry.

But making him feel even more guilty, at that point, serves no one. The disease is already there and he is, sadly, now in need of care. We are now the caregivers and we will do the best we can.

....

Giving care without instilling guilt is a hard chore but I am trying my best to remember that adding guilt to our problems does no good.

The Greatest Gift

How sad when being alive is a living hell. So many people lose their will to live, and perhaps rightfully so, because their level of pain is so terribly high and they have virtually no quality of life left. Our whole day may revolve around controlling their pain and our tears.

We may not be ready for our loved one to die. We haven't had enough time with her yet, we reason. We have more to tell her than time permits.

A very special gift we can give to our loved one is the permission to die when her time comes. Telling our loved one how much we care and that we know how much she hurts, then telling her that it is all right if she is now ready to die — that is possibly the greatest gift we can ever give.

. . . .

Giving the gift of permission cost me more than any other gift I've ever given but I know it was time and I feel content that I did all I could to help during my loved one's life.

AUGUST 30
Not Believing

"I can't believe what you are telling me," we lament to the doctor. "How can you say this is an incurable disease? You are sentencing my mother to death." Our feelings are obvious as we show our disbelief and fear of what is to come.

It is so hard to face the possible death of a person we love; we certainly cannot do it with ease. The very thought of awakening in the morning and knowing our child or parent or sibling or spouse may not be there can make us feel queasy and weak.

In anticipation of what will happen sometime in the future, we try to "make up" for all the wrongs we may have done, to be sure there are no harsh feelings. Then we get on with the business of giving care and love until the end.

....

I don't know exactly why I am so fright-
ened to lose my loved one, yet it seems my
very being is connected to his soul. I pray
I will be able to manage alone.

Loss Of Self-Esteem

So much of who we think we are is based on what we do each day. If we work, our self-esteem is often based on doing a good job, regardless of what job it is. Bringing home a paycheck regularly, rarely missing work, being respectful to other employees and receiving respect in return — these contribute to our feeling good about ourselves. If not for paid work, some people do volunteer work, for we all like to feel good about ourselves.

Suddenly we are called upon to give care to a person we love. We may have to stop working to stay home and give the care. Our self-esteem plummets because we no longer receive praise from anyone and don't feel worthy enough to praise ourselves.

....

Caregiving knocked my sense of self-esteem down until I realized I was doing one of the most important jobs of my life, giving care and help to a person I dearly love. I feel better now.

243

SEPTEMBER 1

Other Causes

It may be tragic to assume incorrectly what another person's health problem is. The elderly are so commonly expected to develop Alzheimer's disease that we sometimes accept lethargy, confusion and loss of memory as the new norm of their lives.

In many cases, there are medical conditions that could be causing the same problems. Be sure the individual gets to a doctor with a responsible adult along to explain the situation.

Thyroid disease, overuse or incorrect use of medicines — especially sleeping pills — as well as depression or alcoholism can cause changes similar to Alzheimer's. Imagine how we would feel if the problem were curable and within a short time we could have the person we have known and loved functioning well on their own.

....

The thought that I might accept as inevitable those health changes which are curable instead of seeking further medical help terrifies me. I am so thankful that my loved one can be helped.

Travel

When a person we love dearly develops a medical problem that requires caregiving, some people go at their new task with a vengeance, cutting themselves off from old friends and from the outside world, except when medical help is required.

It is interesting to note how some caregivers can continue to live their lives, incorporating the needs of the other person into their daily plans. So many times we hear that the two people are planning a trip together. It may take a good bit of advance planning but if both want to go, they pack up and leave.

Long and short vacations and day outings are not prohibitive except in very special cases. Life is meant to be lived, not waiting around for the inevitable to occur.

....

We had more fun on this trip than any other in our lives because we value our relationship so much. We can't wait to go again.

SEPTEMBER 3
Abdicating Care

Some people are just not capable, physically or emotionally, of becoming caregivers. Others are quite capable but choose to hire people so their lifestyle is not interfered with. Each one of us has to do what we need to do.

When professionals, such as doctors or accountants, have a loved one needing care and their own work must go on, *it doesn't mean that they don't love their care recipient*. The caregiver may still be very involved in the care process while not a primary caregiver.

In other sadder cases, the caregiver hires help and never (or rarely) even visits the sick person, who feels deserted. The individual is too busy working, having fun or traveling to even call or stop in. It is a truly sad situation.

....

I feel sorry for those who don't visit their sick loved ones. They lose a marvelous opportunity — one I have been lucky enough to have — of becoming closer than ever to the sick family member.

Visiting

Old friends have called, ones we haven't seen in years. They don't know about the change in our life — that one of us is ill and needs care. What we tell them may well set the pattern for future visits.

Telling the truth is always best, so our old friends don't enter our home expecting everything to be as it was years ago. Let them know in advance what has happened and what to expect.

There is no reason to be embarrassed by something that is beyond our control. What is in our control, however, is how we receive our guests. We may not have homemade cookies ready and the coffeepot on — instant coffee and storebought cookies are fine.

. . . .

People who care about us and whom we care about don't expect us to entertain. They just want to see us and share their time and concern. I thoroughly enjoy their visits.

247

Pets

One of the most unusual prescriptions written by physicians these days is for a kitten, a puppy, a bird or even an aquarium. It has been proven time and time again that people who are elderly, especially if they are alone, have a greater will to live if they have a reason to want to get up each morning.

A kitten or puppy is a compelling reason to get out of bed each day to care for it, to stroke its fur and take it for a walk. People who previously had little interest in life are suddenly eager for each new day to begin.

It is entirely possible that caring for a pet delays the need for caregiving in some cases as pets encourage the individual to get out, be with other people and enjoy life more.

....

I couldn't believe the change when I gave a kitten to my elderly father. I haven't seen him this content for years. And when he is happy, I feel happier, too.

Repulsion

It is not uncommon for family members to be embarrassed by the behavior of loved ones, especially if we are in public and their behavior is inappropriate. Watching a parent or spouse wet themselves or let their nose run can be upsetting even at home.

Embarrassment can easily turn to repulsion if our loved one, not understanding how changed they are by illness, still approach us to make love or to ask for romantic kisses. It is not abnormal to feel repulsed at the very thought of being intimate with an incontinent individual who needs to be fed and bathed.

Repulsion mixes with pity and we are confused and concerned about our ability to be effective caregivers. It is now, repulsed and confused, that we may need to give up the reins, perhaps to a family member, perhaps to a nursing home.

. . . .

In order to survive emotionally myself, I had to stop being the primary caregiver. I had reached overload and I knew it.

249

SEPTEMBER 7

Creating Change

How many times have we heard the phrase, "People cannot change other people. The only person we can change is ourselves." Yet we are often upset by the continual shifts in our home, from bad health to poorer health and back to slightly better health, that we are tempted to try to change our situation a bit.

Bargaining with a person who needs care might work if that person is aware cognitively — but it is still chancy. What right have we to make a person change a whole lifetime of behavior because it suits our lifestyle better?

If communication is possible, then it may help to sit down and talk over the areas of difficulty. Don't be surprised if we are told a thing or two as well! Otherwise we will have to learn to take the good with the bad and deal with life as it is.

....

Giving and accepting care is a two-way street. By discussing our areas of concern we can do justice to this difficult job of caregiving.

Reading Aloud

Reading is a wonderful, quiet hobby that many of us enjoy. While we enjoy reading at our leisure, we may be chagrined to find suddenly that our loved one can no longer handle a book alone.

Reading aloud might amount to setting a short time aside, perhaps for highlights of the morning newspaper or for an afternoon chapter from a book or a new magazine.

Reading aloud can give both people satisfaction. It is a wonderful gift that people who love each other can give to one another. Reading also keeps the mind alert.

. . . .

Both of us feel much more in touch with each other and with current events, as good books help to make us happy and we share this enjoyable activity.

SEPTEMBER 9

The Caregiver's Mood

The attitude of the caregiver can actually affect the attitude of the person to whom they are giving care. When the caregiver has a bad day, it is not uncommon that our recipient also has a bad day as a reflection of our mood.

For this reason it becomes more important than ever that we watch the mood we are in when giving care. If we appear cold and abrupt our care recipient might feel rejected, when the problem is only that we are preoccupied with something entirely unrelated.

Often our care recipient has little contact with other people — in effect, we are sometimes all they have. It helps them if we act pleasantly when giving care, even if we are busy thinking of something else.

....

I know that I get preoccupied when I am doing routine care and sometimes forget to carry on a conversation. I know it will be helpful to my loved one if I remember to be gentle and kind.

Centering Oneself

Losing our sense of self is too easy if we are in a situation where we are required to give care to another person 24 hours a day, seven days each week.

At first we may handle the job easily, not yet recognizing that it may go on for months or even years and that we will become more and more fatigued and short-tempered. It isn't that we mean to have a short fuse but it often happens in a stressful situation.

Spending 10 or 15 minutes alone once or twice a day, just to listen to music or even listen to our own thoughts, is imperative to our daily emotional survival. Without brief pauses to help us remember who we were and who we still are, caregiving would be even more difficult.

. . . .

By centering myself, or only concentrating on me, for a short time each day, I am able to gain back my equilibrium and handle the work that faces me.

SEPTEMBER 11

Advance Grief

What a sad situation it is when we know that the person we love, the person we are caring for 24 hours each day, is soon going to die. Even starting to accept terminal illness can seem impossible.

Whether we know it or not, each and every day we do some grieving, preparing ourselves mentally for the time when our loved one will no longer be with us. This is called advance grieving and it happens often when we are caring for a person who is dying.

In some cases, so much advance grieving is done that when the person does die, it is almost anticlimactic. Other people may have trouble understanding why we are not grieving the way they would expect.

....

There is no right or wrong way to grieve and no one has the right to tell me how to grieve when my loved one dies.

Accidental Abuse

Parents who hit their children or yell at them don't usually mean to, but circumstances and sometimes the child's behavior temporarily push them over the edge. There are many support groups available to help parents deal with their feelings of anger.

Adult caregivers who abuse their care recipients don't usually mean it, but they are so worn out, so overwrought with their ongoing life situation, that sometimes they utter harsh or unkind words and occasionally may even resort to pushing or hitting.

Horrified at what we have done, too ashamed to ask for help or admit it to anyone, we may see the problem escalate and, without knowing it, we have become part of that group of people who abuse helpless elders — the very people we love and are caring for.

. . . .

Just admitting I may have a problem with abuse — verbal or physical — and then going to get help, is the very first step to my recovery.

SEPTEMBER 13

Meditation Connection

When we mention the word meditation, most people conjure up a guru, a climb to a mountain top and a quest for the "real truth" of life. In fact, meditation can be performed and enjoyed at all levels.

Learning to separate ourselves from the stress and hubbub of our days by settling into a deep relaxation may be one of the most important gifts we ever give to ourselves.

For those who have never done relaxation, the simplest way is to find a quiet place, rest our eyes and start to count backward from 500. When we are concentrating on counting, nothing else can enter our minds, and we might even find ourselves floating off a bit — not quite to sleep but to a nice deep state of relaxation.

....

I never thought I would be able to take small relaxation breaks and that if I did, they would be helpful. Now I consider them my mini-vacations and I look forward to each new experience.

Togetherness

Too much togetherness can be the death of some relationships but in the case of caregiver and recipient, it can be a saving grace. People who have had little time for each other may find that being forced to be together is a very special blessing.

At first, having to be together all day long may be difficult. Soon we realize that we can choose to be angry about having to caregive or use the time given us to be with our loved one fruitfully, as a gift to have together.

Talking things over we might not have discussed before, laughing together at situations others might choose to cry over, our relationship continues to grow and our caring for each other is enhanced. How lucky are the people who can take the negative aspects of caregiving and turn them into a positive situation.

. . . .

I consider being asked to caregive an ultimate expression of love and I feel so happy I was chosen.

SEPTEMBER 15
....
Feeling Pain

Most of us have been in the situation of having a sick child, when we would do anything to trade places so we could have their pain. Now that we are caregivers, we may feel the same way, wanting to take the pain away from the person we love or at least share their burden.

It is not our role to take their pain but to offer help and assistance when and where it is needed so that they can deal better with their own illness or pain. Still, in our heart of hearts, when a loved one hurts, we hurt, too.

There is so much we can do that is positive and helpful and we need to remember that. We are giving unselfishly of our love, time and caring. There is no greater gift.

....

I must not let my feelings turn from caregiving to pity for no one wants to be pitied. My role is to be as good a caregiver as I can.

Changing Priorities

It is quite amazing how at different times in our lives, different things are important. For example, a neat, clean house might have been a major priority early in marriage until the children came along. Then most of us noticeably lowered our housekeeping standards, settling for a lesser degree of neatness.

Many folks have a certain idea in their minds about retirement. They plan to travel — sometimes aimlessly — to live a nice life of leisure, going where they wish, when they wish, with the person they love. Wintering in a warm climate is a goal that many share.

Sometimes the need for caregiving cancels our plans, as our loved one is no longer able to travel easily and it may require a great deal of planning to take even a small trip. Wintering in a warm climate may no longer even be an option.

....

I have been able to change priorities all my life and I am capable of changing them once again in order to be a caregiver. I can deal with my disappointment as well.

SEPTEMBER 17

Photo Albums

Sometimes the obvious passes us by, but the caregiving period is a perfect time to sit down with our loved one and label old family pictures so that our children will know years from now who is who. So long as our care recipient is able, talking over old times will be a natural consequence of labeling pictures.

This sounds trivial but it is especially important if our loved one is losing memory, for we may soon be sorry we didn't take the time to label the family pictures while the person's memory was still intact.

Photo albums are a prized possession for most families and often, when asked if they could save one thing from a fire, people say that first they would save the family — then many mention their photo albums.

....

It is painful to look at pictures reminding me of better, happier and healthier days but I know my children will be disappointed if they do not know who all these people are.

Relief

There are all kinds of relief, from the instant type we feel when we use a certain antacid to the kind we feel when we finally know what is really wrong with our loved one — that they are chronically but not terminally ill.

One man likened chronic illness to a lifetime sentence to caregiving — and he was the one in prison. This is a very sad way of looking at the need to caregive since many people manage quite well, continuing to live fruitful and exciting lives, participating in volunteer work and going out with friends.

We also feel a sense of relief when we have established a routine for both of us so each knows what to expect from the other. Knowing our loved one is not going to die — at least not right now — can help us enjoy life.

. . . .

Relief is an understatement of my feelings when I found out my loved one was not going to die. I am also relieved that we get along so well and that I have the privilege of being her caregiver.

SEPTEMBER 19
Secondary Caregiving

For years we managed as a primary caregiver, meeting our loved one's needs and even meeting our own successfully. It was not always easy, but it was a rewarding way to help another person.

Now we are no longer able to give care on a regular basis. Either our health is failing or our loved one's health has changed so much that he can no longer be safely managed at home.

Sometimes the only alternative is a nursing home. While saddened by the decision, we know it is right. Now we move on to functioning as a secondary caregiver, still extremely involved, but not in moment-to-moment decisions.

....

The relief I feel is enormous — but sometimes, unfortunately, so is the guilt. I know there was no other choice so now I will strive to accept this change and get on with life.

Out Walking

Everyone who saw the couple out walking smiled as they passed by. Elderly by anyone's standards, not very strong anymore, they held on to each other, for support and because they were so much in love.

Growing old and frail happens. The role of caregiver may go back and forth, like a hot potato, depending on who needs caregiving the most. But what never changes is how devoted some people are to one another and how obviously they show their love.

For this lucky group of elderly people, caregiving is not a task to be avoided but a cherished act of love that each shares with the other. If only caregiving could be this idyllic for everyone.

....

Blessed be the couple who takes the need for caregiving in stride as an expected part of their last years. I pray that I, too, will be blessed.

SEPTEMBER 21

New Communication

At various times in life we discover that we need new methods of communication. Never are we more aware of that than when our toddlers are just beginning to talk. We love hearing them try to speak and we often mimic their language or at least we talk in simple phrases so they will understand us.

Need for a new kind of communication may also arise if our loved one has suffered a stroke, had a brain tumor or head injury and is having trouble communicating.

Learning new methods of communication, such as word or picture boards, writing notes when speech is difficult or impossible, or using simple gestures can be both helpful and frustrating.

. . . .

If I could choose, I would go back to our old way of communication. But we cannot so I will do the best I can each day to help my loved one.

SEPTEMBER 22
Bring The Mountain

If Mohammed can't come to the mountain, then bring the mountain to Mohammed. This applies to our new lifestyle now that illness and caregiving are part of everyday life.

We both miss being out with people, doing volunteer work, taking part in a book club, quilting, cards or carpentry. If we look hard enough, we can find other people who are also interested in the same hobbies and meetings can be held right in our own homes!

Where there is a will, there is a way. If our care recipient cannot get to the activity, then it is up to us to bring the activity home, so that everyone can participate.

....

Bringing the card-playing club and the book club to our home has altered the course of our lives. Both of us feel happier and more content with our lives now, even if we have to stay at home.

SEPTEMBER 23

Regaining Control

So often severe pain dictates how we live. When the person we are caring for has much pain, it hurts us as well. While it may seem hopeless, there are ways to gain control of one's life by gaining control of pain and pain related behavior.

The physician should be consulted if pain is new or severe for it may be an emergency, and even if it is not, he can help with chronic pain. There are many ways chronic pain can now be helped.

As pain proceeds, self-esteem tends to lower because we have a hard time feeling good about ourselves when our loved one is overwhelmed with pain. By concentrating on what is most important — helping with pain control — we show that we care and are ready to help.

. . . .

Today I will begin helping my loved one deal with pain so that we both can live calmer and more comfortable lives.

Sometimes it seems that it is just too hard to make any plans at all. Now that our loved one is ill and we are having to give care, it is difficult to plan long-term.

Instead if we just take life in small bites, one day at a time, it will be easier and give hope for the future. Planning what will happen just today and then being willing to alter those plans, if necessary, will really help us to deal with today's situation.

By not planning too far ahead we no longer set ourselves up for failure. And if we are finally in a situation where our care recipient's health stabilizes, we can once again begin to make plans — not too distant — but plans that encompass more than one day.

....

Since I was a long-term planner, it has been hard for me to learn to live for the moment. I have learned, however, and I feel proud that we are handling this situation well.

SEPTEMBER 25
Exercise

Just the thought of exercising — or helping our care recipient to exercise — is enough to make us chuckle. How, we wonder, can this person who has been so ill that we have to take care of her, do any exercise?

In fact, there are many kinds of exercise, from simple range-of-motion exercises which can be done alone by the person who is ill or with assistance from the caregiver, to stationary bicycling, using arm pulleys or light wrist and ankle weights while doing mild prescribed exercises.

If it is possible, going to a therapeutic (warm) pool for a supervised exercise program is an excellent idea which both caregiver and care recipient can do together. Exercise is important, as long as it is done regularly, no matter how easy it seems.

....

Being together in the therapeutic exercise program has been most helpful and rejuvenating for us both. I like it and so does my loved one.

Never Too Old

It was obvious the elderly gentleman was depressed. Even people who hadn't known him before the accident could tell by his physical demeanor. His daughter, not young herself, was doing her best to take care of him and cheer him up.

She lived near him and could be with him for a portion of each day. Finally she called their family doctor and described her father's symptoms. "It sounds as though he is depressed. Bring him in and we'll all talk it over." The doctor agreed her father was depressed, gave him an antidepressant and suggested that he begin seeing a psychologist.

"I'm too old for therapy," her father said. But he was wrong. There is no such thing as being too old to benefit from psychotherapy. He did and felt some relief from his symptoms.

....

I never knew the elderly could benefit from therapy. Each day I learn something new and I am grateful there is help for any age.

269

SEPTEMBER 27

Understanding

Nothing is more important about adjusting to one's illness than understanding what has happened to the body and what may happen in the future. Obviously it is important that the caregiver have a full understanding as well.

By better understanding the disease process we will also know better what to expect in the future. Additionally, we may be able to delay some of the inevitable changes by taking extra good care of our loved ones, by following doctor's orders carefully and by making sure our loved one is well fed, well rested and exercised.

This is tough under the best of circumstances but trying to forestall the progression of new symptoms is like trying to stop an avalanche with a child's dump truck. Still, if the physician feels we can help, it is worth our time and trouble.

....

Considering the alternative, anything I can do to help my loved one deal with this ongoing illness, I will do.

As Well As I Can

A defeatist attitude often dominates both the person who is ill or injured and the caregiver. Each person has to work hard on his own state of wellbeing. Each one has to do as well as he can at living this new life — this life that requires care.

When we expect the worst, it is a safe bet the worst will come; but when we expect the best and try hard to keep a strong positive attitude, we have a better chance of doing better, if not physically, at least emotionally.

Illness aside, people who love each other, even if one is ill and the other caregiving, often are happier and better adjusted than those who just don't care or won't show their affection. Love doesn't conquer all but it certainly can help!

. . . .

Attitude can make the difference between our living a miserable life and one in which we both care deeply and don't hesitate to show it.

The Arts

It was the strangest thing. Before Bruce became ill he had no interest in the arts. He was a "man's man," known for his hunting, fishing and skeet-shooting skills. Good old Bruce.

Now he was home after a prolonged hospital stay for a severe first bout with Crohn's disease that necessitated removing part of his colon and using a colostomy bag. Weakened by his illness and with lots of time to think about his life, Bruce came home a new man, not very strong but more patient.

Suddenly he was interested in the arts, even though he could have gone back to some of his old hobbies. He and his wife began to attend concerts — a passion of hers — and he began to paint. When questioned, Bruce simply said, "Life is too precious to waste it killing any of God's creatures."

. . . .

I thank my God I was given a second chance. I now understand the sanctity of marriage and cherish our life together even more than before.

Forgetfulness

The difference between someone who has brain atrophy disease and one with ordinary forgetfulness is that the latter remember that they came into the room for something but can't remember what it was they wanted.

The sick person can't even remember that he was heading into the room. This is a sad illustration of how life changes when a person we love develops Alzheimer's disease or some other brain atrophy disorder.

Adjusting to life as a caregiver with someone who is having memory problems is one of the saddest things of all, for we know what is coming in the future and it is likely to become worse and worse.

. . . .

There is little I can do except offer support and be certain that the person I love so much is safe and well cared for. I am so sad that this has happened to my beloved.

OCTOBER 1
Grandchildren

Many people are elderly by the time the need for caregiving becomes evident. Within this group, some have grandchildren and some may even be lucky enough to have great-grandchildren.

The question often comes up of how the grandchildren will react to obvious physical changes. Grandchildren who are around often are able to draw their own conclusions for they see their grandparent's health change gradually.

Those who see the grandparent less frequently may need a bit more explanation about the illness and how it affects a person. What matters is not that the individual is ill but that she is still blessed with grandchildren who come to visit.

....

Our grandchildren's visits are worth their weight in gold, for they cheer our day and bring an extra measure of joy into our lives.

It has become increasingly common for grown children and their parents to discuss how they want the end of their lives orchestrated if death doesn't come suddenly.

Living Wills are now legal in almost all states. Each person can spell out the most minute details or just make a general statement about what their wishes are, should they be unconscious or unable to make their own decisions.

Living Wills have given many people a sense of control if they should become comatose or mentally incompetent before death. Family members are grateful, too, for the burden of making a decision and praying it is the right one is not theirs.

....

We both felt a remarkable sense of calm once we discussed what had previously been a taboo topic. Now we each know what the other wants and our comfort level for an unknown future has improved.

OCTOBER 3
Talk To Me

It happens, often after that first blissful year of marriage: "You never talk to me the way you used to. I need you to listen to me, to hear what I have to say. I want to know what you are thinking. Please talk to me more."

A lifetime lament for some is not being able to have personal conversations with their marriage partner or parent. People need to talk and people need to be heard.

Sadly, when someone becomes ill and needs a caregiver, often the first things to go are interpersonal relations and casual conversation.

....

Treating my care recipient as I would wish to be treated is a good way for me to begin. It feels, sometimes, as though I am dealing with a person I don't know anymore but I will try to talk more.

Becoming An Advocate

In the beginning of our loved one's need for care we will do almost anything to make sure they are comfortable and that we are following the doctor's orders. After a while, however, things may change and we understand that we cannot do this on a permanent basis.

Perhaps our care recipient has become more ill or is physically more difficult to deal with. Perhaps our own health has deteriorated and we can no longer be primary caregiver. Once other options are explored, the only remaining choice may be nursing home placement.

Having a loved one in a nursing home can be both devastating and a glorious relief. With constant visits and our acting as their advocates, we can be certain they will still get the best of care.

. . . .

Finding the balance between being a pushy relative and asking for reasonable care is difficult but since I am the only one left to protect my loved one, I will be a good but strong advocate.

OCTOBER 5
Hoping

Our inherently human ability to find even the tiniest sliver of hope is the way that many people maintain their personal equilibrium when they are facing physical or emotional ruin. Without hope, there is little or no zest for life.

Everyone who has lost functioning after an accident or injury hopes they will be the exception to the statistics and recover fully. If we are not to recover fully, then we hope for the ability to function on our own.

Hope is what helps us want to awaken each morning. Hope is the undercurrent to all things in our lives — that the flowers will blossom tomorrow — that the sun will shine — that we will be alive to greet the new day — that we can hope for tomorrow.

....

By always being hopeful — even though I am realistic in my hope — I am able to maintain a positive attitude while I assist my loved one.

Real Encouragement

How do we offer encouragement to a person we know is permanently ill and perhaps has a terminal condition? How can we be positive when there is little to be positive about?

These questions and others race around in our minds as we give constant care to our loved one. While there is life, there is reason to feel encouraged.

So long as both people know the truth, that health may not improve or that the illness may be terminal, there is no reason why they can't encourage each other in life's small successes. Encouragement given from the heart is a blessing to the recipient.

. . . .

It was hard at first to find things I could encourage my loved one about until I realized that this was going to be our new lifestyle. Once I accepted that fact, giving encouragement got easier.

OCTOBER 7

Apologies

Everyone knows how hard it can sometimes be to apologize, especially if we don't feel we have done anything wrong. It's remarkable how many caregivers mention that no matter what they do for their care recipients, they are criticized.

In fact, this isn't really the type of criticism that needs a response but simply the way in which our loved one is expressing fear and discomfort at having to be taken care of. No apologies are needed, for this situation is no one's fault.

Certainly, if there is something we are being legitimately criticized for, we should talk it over and change our behavior. But in most cases, the criticism comes from sadness and discontent — not with us but with the situation.

....

Few people I know ever wanted to have a family member taking care of them. My loved one hates being cared for but we are both trying to make the best of this situation.

Lonely And Scared

Before the need for caregiving became evident, our loved one may have tried, as many elderly people do, to take care of himself. This became harder and harder and soon was too much.

By using outside services such as Meals On Wheels and grocery shopping services, the elderly person successfully stayed at home — alone. However, he was getting more lonely and more and more scared about his failing health.

When a health change occurs often suddenly as from a stroke, a fall or a heart attack, the elderly may no longer be able to stay home alone and care for themselves. Now the time has come to accept caregiving and while they might not like it, they are not as frightened and lonely any more.

. . . .

I know it was terribly sad for my parent to give up his independence and accept my care so I will try my best to be a caregiver without being intrusive in his life.

OCTOBER 9
Reconciling Life

Few people are ever ready for life to end. We hear stories about people who are not finished with their projects, who always have more to do, more life to live. Yet when it is evident they are going to die, many make their peace and quietly leave this world.

Now the situation is entirely different. It is not the coming of death that we reconcile to but the quality of the life that remains — a life that is now dramatically different from the one we anticipated for our loved one. In our heart of hearts we had hoped our parent or spouse could stay independent, take care of their own needs — that was their fervent desire as well.

Now everyone has to reconcile to a new kind of life — one that may be just as fruitful and valuable — but one in which the individual needs to accept care from another person.

. . . .

Accepting care from another person is not easy. I will do my best to ensure that care is given with the utmost respect.

OCTOBER 10
Softening The Truth

When is it right to avoid telling the whole truth about an individual's changing medical condition? These situations are so individual that each one must be decided according to the needs of the person asking about it.

If it is a small child, for example, who asks, "Why does Grammy act like that?" — "Why does Grammy have to sit in that wheelchair?" — an answer can be given that is not complete but geared to the child's level of understanding.

"Grammy's legs are weak, so she needs to sit in the wheelchair," or "Grammy is sick and has trouble remembering," are more than adequate answers for small children, who can only absorb so much information and should only be told what they can understand.

....

Softening the truth for a child is not a lie but a gently offered gift. As the child grows older, I will give more specific answers.

OCTOBER 11

Understanding Friends

There is no feeling like the one we have when we think we are completely alone. This feeling of aloneness may happen many times in life. We may feel entirely alone when we have been blessed with our first baby. Joy was what most of us anticipated; a sense of loneliness is what we got.

As newly divorced or widowed people, we can be overwhelmed with loneliness, and it is often our dear — or even new — friends who pull us through the hard times.

Now our loved one is ill and we are the caregiver. Once again, we may feel overwhelmed and lonely. Understanding friends, people we have shared our feelings with for years, people we trust implicitly, can help pull us through one of life's toughest challenges.

....

It was hard to trust anyone with the feelings I am experiencing but no one censured or condemned me. They just let me talk and they understood my feelings. I am very lucky to have such good friends.

Recovery

We were finally used to the new caregiving role. In fact, many of us willingly gave up a job to be there when our loved one needed us. Now our patient has recovered from the accident, injury or surgery and may not need our care any more.

What do we do now? Our entire day, in fact our entire life plan, had shifted over and been accepted as caregiving. Of course, we are happy our loved one is well again, but we feel left behind in the dust and we are not sure how to handle the rest of our lives.

Do we go back to work? Should we look for a new job or perhaps retire? We never expected to be the one who was left at home, who was left behind. This takes some serious thought as we decide our future.

. . . .

I didn't mean it maliciously yet I hoped to continue caregiving so I would feel important. I am glad he is better but I am confused about my feelings. I can start again but I'm not sure how.

Journals For Balance

How difficult it can be to care entirely for another human being's needs! If their need were less, if we had time for ourselves, things would be different. But we are consumed with their needs and there is little time left for us.

Journal writing can be a wonderful outlet for these pent-up feelings. Even if we have never written a word before, this is a way to describe secret and very private feelings that no one ever need see. Since we can receive no feedback or criticism from the journal itself, it is very safe to write down our thoughts.

Not all thoughts will be negative, yet whatever we are thinking, this private journal gives us a place to unburden, a chance to talk to the pages as if we were talking to a beloved friend.

. . . .

At first I felt strange writing down my thoughts, especially since I rarely have expressed them out loud. Soon I realized how important it was to my wellbeing. Now I do it daily.

Macho Males

How difficult it must be for a man who used to be so macho, such a high-powered executive, to realize that he is ill with a disease so serious that he will soon need care.

This can happen with illnesses like Lou Gehrig's disease, terminal cancer or a brain atrophy disease such as Alzheimer's. The hardest part for the person who is ill is accepting that the physicians have told the truth and he will likely go downhill quickly.

For those of us who care for such a person, we have to expect to be given orders at first, for that individual is certain he knows how best to direct care. As the illness gets worse, we begin to do it our way, the easiest way, for his judgment will diminish as his health continues to deteriorate.

. . . .

It was so hard when my husband gave me orders about how to care for him, especially since I gave up my job to do it. Now I understand he was trying to hold on to his pride and I feel so sad.

OCTOBER 15

Reversing Roles

Even when we are really good at caregiving, we do sometimes get sick ourselves — the flu, a strained back or a bad cold. Then we don't know what to do. Do we call someone in for help? Do we try to manage on our own?

What a surprise it is when our loved one, the person we are caring for, tries to help us get better. In some cases, this works fine, especially if the care recipient only needs help with bathing and dressing. If he really can't care for himself but still wants to help us feel better, it is a very warm feeling although we may fear that he might do something dangerous, like spilling hot water.

There is a special feeling when the person we are caring for makes us tea or toast. They are, for the short term, showing their love for us by trying to help us get better.

....

I was so touched when my loved one, who can barely manage to walk on his own, brought me tea and toast. It reminds me how special he really is.

288

Showing Love

The experience of caregiving is not a negative one for many people. "I wouldn't have it any other way," remarked Helen at her caregiver's support group. "But I admit that I get awfully tired and need some time away from my sister. She can be so annoying — but then she always could! We still fight just the same as we used to when we were kids, but that doesn't mean I don't love her."

So many people feel the same way while caregiving for a relative, close friend or spouse. This is, they are convinced, the way we can show our love and appreciation. Not all of us agree, since some of us are too dragged down physically and mentally by the physical work of caregiving. But we do agree that giving care to a person we love is the ultimate expression of love.

....

I am more than willing to do the caregiving and probably would have done it without being asked. I love this person enough to subjugate my life in order to give care.

289

OCTOBER 17

Dangerous Times

For just a few moments Jack allowed himself the luxury of closing his eyes and taking a 10-minute catnap. He awakened to a pounding on the door. It was a neighbor with his wife in tow and she was completely nude! Jack was embarrassed, more that he had fallen asleep than her state of undress, for everyone knew she was suffering from Alzheimer's.

A few days later it happened again. Jack was in the bathtub and his wife was asleep. The next thing he knew the fire alarms went off; somehow she started a fire in her bedroom.

Jack knew then that they were playing with danger and that she would need to be placed in a facility where she could not endanger herself. He found a very fine nursing home and placed her there where he knew she would be safe.

....

No matter how hard I tried, I couldn't watch my wife every second. When things started getting dangerous, I knew I couldn't let my foolish pride keep her at home any longer. She is safe now.

Reaction

Alice took sleeping pills, prescribed because she had trouble sleeping since she was alone.

Before long, her health deteriorated, and a neighbor was stopping in every day to make meals, clean up and help Alice with her bath. Several mornings the neighbor found evidence that Alice had been cooking food during the night but didn't remember that she had.

A few weeks later she could not fully awaken Alice one morning, so she called Alice's doctor and took her to his office. Alice had figured that if one sleeping pill was good, then two were better. Her overuse of the pills had nearly caused a serious problem. The doctor, not knowing how ill Alice was, kept refilling the prescription without requiring a visit.

....

I felt awful telling the doctor. Now a nurse comes and stays with her. I feel guilty for taking away her independence but I know it is not my fault.

OCTOBER 19
....
Drinking Loneliness Away

Homer had recently lost his wife of 70 years. Sarah had been the joy of his life, the mother of his children and the glue that kept the family together. He missed her desperately.

Evenings came and Homer didn't know what to do with himself. This was the time when he and Sarah used to talk. So he took a little drink. Before long he was taking little drinks all day long.

Drinking took away Homer's loneliness. In fact, he was never lonely — instead he was just drunk. Unfortunately, Homer fell into a new and very prevalent pattern, that of elderly adults who become alcoholics. His family quickly realized what was happening and he got appropriate treatment, which doesn't often happen. Homer soon found other ways to keep himself busy.

....

I am still lonely, but I know now I dare not drink to assuage my loss. I am in an adult daycare program and some other activities and I am much happier.

Looking Normal

Appearances mean everything to some people. Even with the best of intentions, some caregivers aren't able to handle it well when the person for whom they are caring either looks or acts strangely or inappropriately, at home or in public.

If our loved one is very ill, we would not think of criticizing or correcting, for it cannot be helped. But just as a parent is embarrassed when an exhausted toddler has a temper tantrum in the grocery store, so we are sometimes embarrassed by our loved one's behavior.

Just knowing that we feel embarrassed makes us feel awful. We wonder what is wrong with us, the caregiver? Here we are, knowing full well that our care recipient is not acting this way on purpose, but it still bothers us.

. . . .

I feel so guilty that I look for excuses to get out alone, to leave my loved one at home. I need time to be away from a very difficult problem and I am granting myself that time.

OCTOBER 21
Being Scared

For dozens of years the couple has been together, through good times and bad, through bickering and quiet times, through sickness and in health and now back to the final sickness.

Willingly we give care, for we would have it no other way, yet something gnaws at us all the while. "How will I function without this marvelous person who has been part of my life for so long?" we wonder. Feeling scared of what we know is inevitable, we are nearly paralyzed with sadness.

There is nothing we can do but live in the moment — giving care as it is needed, and put aside our own fear for the time being. Grief support groups and those for caregivers are there if we can attend them and they will help us. Otherwise, we just will have to await the inevitable.

. . . .

I cannot imagine life without my spouse. Even though we have had some rough times, we have always been in love. I will love her always, even when she is gone.

A New Career

Never once did it occur to her not to care for her younger sister, who was dying of cancer. She loved her sister dearly and wouldn't leave her alone in this time of need. What she didn't know is how significantly it would change her future.

Instead of being fatigued, she was invigorated by the need to be needed. When her sister did die, a few months later, the caregiving sister had her home certified as a foster home for elderly adults.

Three older people moved in, all of whom needed supervision, but none of whom needed total care. She was so happy with her new little household, cooking, cleaning and never, ever being lonely any more. The families of her three boarders were delighted and so was she. Imagine, a whole new career in her 70s.

....

I never dreamed that caring for my sick sister would give me a whole new chance at life, at being with other people, at feeling so good about myself. I am so lucky.

12 Steps

Just becoming a caregiver does not mean that we have led lives pure as the driven snow. Each caregiver brings along the sum and total of all life experiences, both good and bad.

If substance abuse or co-dependency has been part of a caregiver's background, and the caregiver has been involved in a 12-Step group, he should do everything possible to keep up with his commitment, even if it means hiring someone to come in and take his place at home for a few hours each week.

Maintaining something as crucial as a 12-Step program, especially while caregiving, when our defenses are likely to be down, is one of the most important gifts we can give to ourselves.

....

Just because I am responsible for someone else's care right now does not mean I should ignore my own needs. I am important, too, and I can take good care of myself.

Hope

As we step into the role of caregiver, we realize that we are unwilling to give up the hope that our loved one's health will improve soon. Hope is so uniquely human. Hope offers us a chance.

Whether the move into full-time caregiving is gradual or we have already been doing some of it and are now doing more, still we cling to the hope that things will soon get better and our loved one can resume a normal life, the old life, without needing a caregiver.

When a human being gives up hope, we recognize that as the beginning of the end. Most people will fight to survive, hoping against hope that a miracle cure or surgery will be discovered even at the end of their lives. Most people never stop hoping.

. . . .

While there is life, there is hope. I intend never to give up hope that things will improve and that my loved one will live a bit longer.

297

OCTOBER 25

Volunteering

So many generous people volunteer these days that our president calls volunteers "a thousand points of light." Even while working full-time jobs and raising children, so many people still find the time to do at least some volunteer work.

Once we are full-time caregivers, however, our time is no longer our own — at least not wholly. Surprisingly, people feel guilty when they have to say no when asked to volunteer. So they have found alternate ways to fulfill themselves and help others.

These unselfish folks offer to bake for the school bake sale, so long as someone can stop by and pick up their cakes and cookies. They make spaghetti for the church pot-luck supper. Others knit, crochet or do woodwork for organizations to give as door prizes.

. . . .

Once a volunteer, always a volunteer. While my time is not my own these days, I still have enough time left to help other people.

Cooler Weather

Depending upon where one lives, the end of October usually heralds the beginning of cold weather. Often the leaves have blown off the trees and we know snow is soon to follow.

What a wonderful time to bundle up our loved one and go for a ride or a walk around the neighborhood. People who are house-bound because of illness miss getting out. Late October is a wonderful time to take a drive, even if it is just to the local coffee shop.

If our care recipient has special needs, it might be best to go during an off-time, when the coffee shop will not be crowded, so we can explain what those needs are or take care of them ourselves. Perhaps a bib or hot chocolate cooled by milk are the ticket, but the "trip" out of the house will be appreciated and everyone will feel better.

. . . .

It must be very confining to go out only rarely. Seeing the joy in my loved one's face when I proposed a ride for cocoa, I vowed to do it more often. We both had fun.

Blame

"I'm not a very good caregiver," we may think. "I was just not cut out for this job." Some people may have no problem doing it but many feel a sense of betrayal that their loved one became ill and subsequently took away their freedom.

Even when we are giving care willingly and with love, things happen in the course of care. Our loved one may fall and sustain a cut that needs stitches or get burned on a hot cup of coffee. Bedsores may develop no matter how hard we try to keep them at bay or the illness may get worse.

It's amazing how much personal shame we place upon ourselves, and personally accept the blame for — if we feel we have not done the job to the absolute best of our ability.

. . . .

Unless there is real neglect, we are doing the very best we can. Blaming ourselves only serves to make us feel guilty. It does nothing but make us feel bad.

A Better Way

There is no one way to be a caregiver, no rule book that shows us how to act and what to do. At first we may stumble in our new job, feeling inadequate as we grope our way through the tasks.

Before too long it becomes second nature and even if we don't much like having to give care, we now know how to do the job. Bathing a 200-pound man seemed impossible at first but now I have learned the best way to do it.

Soon we begin to find shortcuts, ways to make our job easier. Some we learn ourselves from trial and error, others we pick up from sharing at a caregivers' support group. Each of us has our own way to caregive and we can take the best ways of others, add our ideas and create a unique style of caregiving.

. . . .

I realized recently that I have begun to apply some sound principles of business and physics to caregiving. It makes my job easier and now we are both happier.

OCTOBER 29
Serenity Self-Care

One wouldn't naturally associate the word caregiver with the term serenity. However, in this very difficult job of being a caregiver, we need to look to those things which cause us to feel serene. There is more at stake here than just our loved one's health.

Also at stake is our health, all facets of it, the physical, the emotional, the spiritual. Unless we are at peace with ourselves, we will not know serenity.

For this reason, it is crucial that we take care of our inner — our spiritual — needs as well as our outer health. We need a place to go — not necessarily away from the house — within ourselves, to worship in whatever way we wish and yes, even to praise ourselves for the work we are doing.

....

*Feeling peaceful and serene is part of how
I survive as a worthwhile human being.
I am doing important work, both in looking after someone else and taking care of
my own needs.*

Compromising

All through adulthood we have had to compromise. Not all of us got everything we wished for or had life go the way we wished but we learned that if we were willing to compromise a bit, we would likely still find happiness.

Now we have to compromise in a wholly different way. We are taking care of another person's needs, to a lesser or greater extent, depending upon how ill they are. They will certainly have opinions about their personal care and so will we.

Only by talking together, if that is possible, can we decide together the best way to accomplish all the tasks which come with caregiving. Each person has the right to express an opinion. Where we can compromise, we should. It is a small thing to do.

....

I am not so stubborn that by compromising I can't make my loved one's care a bit easier. It is hard for both of us but talking together will help us understand one another's needs.

OCTOBER 31
Halloween

Unless we live in an area where there are no children, we can expect this late afternoon and evening to be interrupted with the ringing doorbell and happy shouts of "Trick or Treat!"

We remember well how exciting going out on Halloween night used to be and so we prepare for the children by purchasing some candy or apples and by designing and carving a pumpkin to light their way. What joy and wonder the youngest ones show and what a delight it is to feel a part of their excitement!

It would have been just as easy to turn out our lights and ignore the children but we both want to participate as much as possible in life, in joy and in watching the happiness of children as we open our door to them.

. . . .

I remember so well all the years we trick-or-treated, the homemade costumes, the candy we couldn't wait to eat and bobbing for apples. It's fun to watch others having such fun.

NOVEMBER 1

The Microwave

For the 55 years of their marriage, Joshua's
wife did all the food preparation, always having
meals hot on the table when he arrived home
from work. He could depend upon her. She
always had a hot delicious dinner for him.

Now she was depending upon him more and
more. Since her stroke, she needed total care
and he was the one who was there to give it.
The only problem, the thing he worried about,
was how to prepare meals — he didn't even
know how to brew a cup of tea.

His children stepped in and bought him a
microwave. Then they took him to the grocery
store and showed him the nutritious food for
every meal that were available for microwaving.
Every now and again they brought over frozen
meals from their homes. He learned how to use
the microwave to prepare those, too.

. . . .

*I am very proud of myself. For an old
man, I quickly learned something new
and now I can take care of our needs.*

NOVEMBER 2

Respecting Rights

Some people mistakenly think that needing a caregiver takes one's personal rights away. Nothing could be further from the truth. In fact, if the individual is lucid and cooperative, this is especially the time when they need to express feelings and have their rights respected.

Siblings who care for one another, spouses who wouldn't think of letting any other person do this job and parents who are caring for an ill adult child understand the importance of maintaining dignity and respecting rights.

Respecting the other person's rights might take many forms, from asking their opinion to talking about the events of the day. Even people who can barely talk understand that their rights are being respected and they are grateful to be able to maintain their dignity.

....

I wondered how I would do as a caregiver since my natural impulse would be either to not talk at all or to talk in baby talk. I quickly learned that speaking normally, with respect, works best.

NOVEMBER 3
Having A Party

"How about having a party?" Nathaniel asked his wife Nina. She looked at him as if he were crazy. He knew she was wondering why. He explained, "The people who love you have always loved you in spite of your multiple sclerosis. A lot of people would like to see you."

Unhappily Nina agreed. Nate went about doing all the invitations. He asked everyone to bring something to share. They were all delighted to have the opportunity to visit — the old group was back together once again.

Nina was at the door in her wheelchair, skeptical but excited. She hadn't realized how much she had missed her friends as they hugged and kissed her. They partied for hours, talked over old times and they all had a wonderful evening.

....

We just had not realized how we had let Nina's illness tuck us away into a private and tiny closet. Last week we opened ourselves up to friends and now both feel like petals on a newly blooming flower.

307

NOVEMBER 4

Theme Dinner

Remember the ancient days — the days when we were teenagers and very young adults? Nothing was more exciting then than being with friends and having a party.

If we try, we can still have some of that same excitement. What about planning a theme dinner with your loved one, doing the shopping together and preparing it together as well? Realistically it may mean we prepare and our care recipient keeps us company but at least both of us are doing it together.

How about an Italian dinner or Nouvelle Cuisine? Maybe Czechoslovakian would be fun, or perhaps it is southern food the two of us decide upon. What matters is having fun together and having something different to look forward to.

. . . .

Every Tuesday we have a theme — or special request dinner. Sometimes I choose and sometimes my loved one does but most often we decide together. Anticipating Tuesday is fun all week.

308

No Condescension

All one has to do is go into a local shopping mall and watch people who are with others less healthy than themselves. Some are pushing wheelchairs with pride, obviously happy about where they are and who they are with.

Others are obviously nasty and condescending. "I wish you would sit up, Mother," one may remark, while another admonishes, "But I told you to go before we left the house!"

It hurts us to see other people, especially the elderly and small children, being treated in such a way. It is apparent what other people think about it, too.

. . . .

Our situation may be hard but it never merits being unkind. I will work at remembering every day to treat my loved one as I would wish to be treated.

NOVEMBER 6
Pride In Work

When we were in the work force, most of us had pride in our jobs. Whether we were instrumental in building a skyscraper, designing it, keeping it clean or being a supplier of goods, we felt personal pride.

In any job we had, at any level, it was important to care about our work, about how we presented ourselves to other people, and especially how we were rated on the job.

Now that our job has changed so radically, we are both boss and sole employee. Caregiving is very hard work. Generally, the only one who sees our work is us. Yet no job, except raising children, has ever been so important.

....

It was difficult to give up my work at first until I realized that I wasn't leaving the job market, I was just moving to a far more crucial position.

Planning Weekends

Just because we are now in a situation in which one person is giving some care to another does not mean that there should not be any fun or special events to plan for together.

One time we can plan together is the weekend. Do we both like movies, for instance, but find it too hard to go to see one? Renting a movie and viewing it together is fun. Make a batch of popcorn and enjoy.

Friends might be invited over for a simple meal or dessert on Saturday evening or just to visit. What matters is that we not give up looking forward to the future, the near as well as the distant future.

....

We have sequestered ourselves too much these past few months. It is time for us to accept the medical challenges life has handed us and move on. Planning special times together will help us begin again.

NOVEMBER 8
Special Meals

Some people like tapioca and some despise it. Others thrive on eggs, any kind, any style, any time. Some love pot roast, while others prefer chicken a la king. Individual tastes differ.

Somehow, now that our loved one is ill, we may be in the habit of preparing food methodically, without giving any thought to the preference of the person we are caring for. This isn't fair, one more sad fact of life.

Think, instead, about either shopping together for a special meal or setting up a "choice" day for each of you. Perhaps Tuesdays and Sundays might be the days each one gets to choose the meal. It is a small thing but when there is little to look forward to, it makes time move a bit more quickly.

....

By offering a choice in meals and being willing to take the time to discuss preferences, we both have something special to look forward to. This is a small gesture, one I can easily handle.

NOVEMBER 9
Exploring

How often we hear that native New Yorkers don't ever visit their city's landmarks. They live all their lives in a wonderful mecca of culture and fascinating places and never take the time to visit any of them.

The same is true for most people. They live for years in one geographical area, know there is a historic sight, a public house or a lovely garden, but don't ever take advantage of what the home area has to offer.

By planning small trips for two or three hours — after checking to be sure they are accessible and appropriate — we can build some excitement and a wonderful opportunity to learn and have fun into our lives.

....

It takes so little effort to go on small day trips or to visit local historical or interesting points. I am happy for both of us that we have decided to do some exploring. It makes life exciting.

NOVEMBER 10
A Picnic For Two

_While we are thinking about day trips and local sights of interest, why not take along a homemade picnic breakfast, lunch or dinner? We have a tendency to forget how much fun it is to eat food we have prepared ahead, especially foods we love, like fried chicken or even simple peanut butter and jelly or bologna sandwiches.

Certainly it may not be a blanket at the beach but there are park benches and other appropriate areas where two people — even if one of them is mobility impaired — can enjoy a picnic meal together.

....

Along with our food, I remembered to bring along a favorite tape and we had lovely background music with our food. We both felt good about getting out and eating in a totally different surrounding.

Re-evaluating Needs

When there are health issues, there is often an initial visit from a nurse or a physical therapist to see what the care recipient is going to need in the way of services. This is crucial when setting up the support team, which of course includes the caregiver.

Too often that initial consultation is the only one that is done. Not taken into consideration is the fact that our loved one may be getting worse, and now needs more care, some of which we cannot give.

We need to take matters into our own hands by phoning the physician, explaining the changes and requesting a new evaluation for outside services. Most doctors will cooperate and set the wheels in motion for a re-evaluation.

. . . .

It hurts me to admit that my loved one is getting weaker or more ill but I understand the importance of being sure that the right services are available to optimize both my care and medical care.

315

NOVEMBER 12

Arranging The Room

People tend to be creatures of habit, and one habitual attitude is that the bedroom is the bedroom, even if it is upstairs and very inconvenient. We keep trying to use it the same way we always did.

Now it is time to look at our living quarters with different eyes. Would it be better, now that our loved one is ill, to arrange for a hospital bed and privacy screen in the dining room or living room? Could a portable commode be brought in to facilitate toileting?

Being in the midst of things instead of tucked away in a bedroom most of the time can lift a person's spirits and make the days much more pleasurable for everyone. Of course, we will have to put up with more mess but that isn't important right now.

....

I do like to keep things in order but when I put myself in my loved one's place, I realized how much nicer it would be to face a window, be able to visit easily with friends and enjoy each day.

Memory Lane

Older people especially enjoy taking trips down memory lane, talking about the old days, the times when they were kids and about their earlier life in general. If we have a loved one who is suffering from a brain atrophy disease such as Alzheimer's, that portion of memory may be all that is left intact.

All we hear from them are the old stories because so many can't remember or understand what is happening today. This may be frustrating, especially when the person cannot remember how to go to the bathroom alone.

Perhaps it would help if we took the time to record some of the stories. Hearing them from the mouth of one who was there could be a wonderful gift to future generations.

. . . .

When I realized how frustrating it was to hear the old stories so often, I decided to record them. Now we are doing something valuable for future generations of our family.

NOVEMBER 14
Power Of Attorney

There may come a time, especially if we have elderly parents in failing health who live far away, that we will need to get a durable power of attorney. This may be very important to protect our parents financially.

It is very hard to accept that our parent, the person we always could depend upon, can no longer manage her own household accounts. Being able to do it for that parent at long distance can mean the difference between needing a nursing home or having her stay at home in a familiar setting.

As our parents become less capable, we are likely to feel the strain of trying to be a long distance caregiver. In some cases it might be easier to hire someone to move in or at least be there a few hours a day. This will bring us some peace of mind.

....

I hate seeing my parent grow old and incapable of making personal decisions. I am trying to adjust to the possibility of losing a parent but it is very hard to do.

NOVEMBER 15

Conservator

There is another, often more convenient, way to handle the issue of money and one's aging parent at long distance. That is to arrange for an individual or a conservatorship company nearby to be hired or court-appointed for your parent.

One should investigate this company or individual first, making sure they are bonded and well-known in their geographic area. It might be wise to have a lawyer arrange this important task.

Also, we should always receive copies of all transactions in order to keep track of our parent's funds. This enhances our peace of mind and guarantees us that money is only being spent as it should be. There is always a monthly fee for a conservator.

. . . .

After I looked over the disarray of my parent's financial condition, I realized I couldn't handle it long distance. The conservatorship has worked wonders in quelling my fears and helping my parents.

NOVEMBER 16

A Special Service

In the last several years a brand new service is being offered in many large cities: qualified groups oversee the wellbeing of aged and ill people.

For a fee, they will do those chores that we would do if we lived nearby. They check on the aging adult, make sure there are groceries and that meals are prepared, perhaps giving some care as well. This is not a full-time aide but a service that oversees through various employees, all the needs of our aging or ill parents.

It is wise to check either with the Attorney General's office or with the local governmental branch that works with senior citizens to be certain you are hiring a reputable group.

....

The relief I felt when I knew my parent would be well cared for without my having to drive 500 miles each weekend is definitely measurable. I am more relaxed and comfortable now.

Praise

It is the rare caregiver who takes on the job for praise. After all, when one is cleaning the toilet bowl after our care recipient misses again, wiping up spilled lemonade and trying to grab some sleep when our loved one sleeps — each and every day — it certainly isn't done for praise.

Yet wouldn't it be lovely if a family member or close friend took the time to remember the caregiver, to offer a few hours off once in a while, or even remembered to say thank you. Caregiving is often a thankless job.

Even close family members, brothers and sisters or adult children, forget how hard we are working. How nice it would be to be relieved for a while or given some praise.

....

Caregiving, especially now that my loved one is so childlike, is a sad and thankless job. I have never worked so hard at any other job before and I am extremely proud of myself and the job I am doing.

NOVEMBER 18

Dressing Up

When we don't feel well, if we have the flu or a bad cold, it is easier to stay in our night-clothes and to put on a bathrobe for meals or when we step outside to get the paper.

This pattern would be easy for us to fall into for our care recipient as well. After all, they are unwell and constantly spilling or soiling their clothes. Staying in nightclothes, however, just isn't a good idea. For one thing, our loved one might be confused about whether it is day or night.

More important, however, is that each person needs to maintain his pride and personal dignity and staying in pajamas or a nightgown is one way of indicating that what one wants or how one feels is not important.

. . . .

Even though my loved one is confused and disoriented, it is important that I keep him dressed and clean. This not only is important to him but it makes me feel better, too.

Getting A Job

Herschel's whole family was stunned when Shirley, his wife of 35 years, decided to get a job after two years of non-stop caring for him. She explained, "As times goes on and he understands less and less. I am more frustrated and angry with him.

"I think the only way to preserve my sanity and keep him safe is for me to be gone several hours a day. All the money I make will be spent to pay a replacement person to care for him but it will be worth every penny."

Shirley understood that she had to make a change and she was doing it. She not only knew that her husband was hard to care for but she sensed that her anger at his illness was getting out of hand. Since no one else offered to help, she decided to help herself.

. . . .

Getting a job was the smartest thing I ever did. I met another woman who was also caring for her husband and we became fast friends. I look forward to work and am far less angry now.

323

NOVEMBER 20
Wanting To Die

Nature may be cruel sometimes and a person who has a terminal illness may suffer for months before death comes. The worst problem can surface when that person repeatedly begs the caregiver, "Please, help me die. I can't live this way any more."

Hospice programs can be arranged right at home to assist with pain control and to help dying people tie up the loose ends of their lives.

Even when there is an in-home hospice program in place, our loved one may still beg us, not understanding the possible criminal implications, but just wanting to be out of misery. A Living Will would be a good idea, if it hasn't already been signed. Dying is scary for everyone but offering assistance, other than comfort, is really not a viable option.

....

There were plenty of times when I was tempted to help my loved one die but in my heart of hearts I just couldn't consider it an option. It hurts me to say it now but I am comfortable with my choice.

Surrounded By Family

In the best of cases, caregiving is a family affair. A schedule is arranged for each adult child to come in and help the parent who is caregiving or just to come in if there is no other person to caregive.

In this way, the entire family not only shares the burden and the joys of caregiving but each has a better sense of what is going on and how hard it is for the other family members.

Sharing may be arranged in another way, with one person doing all the cooking during the week for both caregiver and recipient. Another does the grocery shopping and a third cleans the house. Perhaps grandchildren might mow the lawn and shovel snow.

. . . .

When caregiving is a family affair, no one person has to shoulder the full burden. We all feel better when we can share in this effort.

NOVEMBER 22
Outside Visitors

Too often, when we are in a caregiving situation, and especially if our loved one is becoming more childish, we tend to discourage visits from outside people, even people who know us well.

Perhaps we let the minister or rabbi visit occasionally but we may feel uncomfortable with others seeing our loved one acting the way we see them. We tend to get more reclusive, letting only family members in, ashamed of our loved one's behavior.

Old friends want to share our pain. They are not just coming to see our loved one but to offer their emotional and spiritual support to us, for they understand how difficult the job of caregiving is. It is hard to let others see our pain but once we do, we know how much it helps and we are usually glad we did.

. . . .

I forget, sometimes, that I used to have an active social life, too. Now that I am willing to be with friends again, my life has opened up and the caregiving tasks seem just a bit easier.

Still Hoping

The human spirit never ceases to amaze. Even when we know our loved one has a terminal disease, we hope, until they draw their very last breath, that a miracle will happen.

Without hope, life would not be worth living. When we are poor, we hope for money or a better job. When we have no children, we hope to have a family. Now we want a miracle.

When there is illness — either ours or that of a loved one — we hope that we will be the exception and beat it, recovering and moving back into normal life. We may know in our hearts this will not happen but we continue to hope anyway.

....

To give up hope would be to give up on life. In order to keep myself going as a caregiver, I need to hope that tomorrow will be better, that I will get through this intact. Hope holds me together.

NOVEMBER 24

Dying At Home

How sad we feel now that the person we have cared for all this time, our wonderful loved one, is near the end of life. Perhaps we have had a discussion in which she asked to die at home.

An in-home hospice or the family's physician can put in place any equipment or special services that are needed. Hospice care helps those who want to die at home do so with grace and dignity.

We may feel squeamish about having our loved one die at home. Uncertain how we are going to handle it, we agree to it since that is to be their last wish. Most people say it is a lovely experience, that they feel peace as the death draws near.

....

Dying is only one breath away from life and people have the right to die where they choose. I am happy I agreed to let my loved one die at home, surrounded by familiar things and family members.

Not Selling Out

There may come a time when there is no choice but to place our loved one in a nursing home. This may happen because it is no longer safe at home, because our health is falling apart rapidly or because we can no longer physically cope.

To some, placing a loved one in a nursing home feels like selling out, as though we are breaking a sacred promise that we never should have agreed to in the first place. This is not selling out; it is looking for the best care when home care is no longer an option.

Certainly we have our own feelings to deal with but we recognize — now that he is away from home — how frail and disoriented our loved one has become, that he doesn't even know he is in a nursing home.

....

My heart ached the day I took my mother to the nursing home but I soon realized that she was as happy there as at home. I am still her caregiver but in a different way. I made a good decision.

NOVEMBER 26

Roasting The Turkey

At the end of November comes Thanksgiving, a holiday many of us hold near and dear to our hearts. Whether from a nursing home or a board-and-care facility, many of us choose to bring our loved one home for the big meal.

It is a joy, even if she is confused, to know that we are bringing a loved one home for Thanksgiving dinner. If the person is a bit confused or disoriented, be certain to explain to the small children that they may not be recognized, and why.

Assign a family member to do the pick-up and bring the sick person to the house. No more than two to three hours should be allotted for the visit as the person will tire easily and ask to "go home" — meaning the nursing home.

. . . .

When my loved one first asked to "go home," I felt shattered when I realized that "home" meant the nursing home. Now I am delighted that we all spent time together and that the visit itself went well.

330

Denying The Truth

Sometimes facing the truth is just too hard. We choose instead to delude ourselves, to tell ourselves that this caregiving situation is only temporary, that our loved one will recover soon.

In some lucky cases this is true, as after an automobile accident or when a loved one is recovering from a heart attack or from surgery. More often that not, however, we can expect the course of our care recipient's health to deteriorate. More and more care will be needed as the months pass.

Eventually we do have to face the truth — that our loved one's health will never be restored. Facing the truth hurts, for it means we will never have that person back the way he was before. Now we have an entirely different person to care for and love.

. . . .

I tried to deny the truth, yet I could see it before my eyes. I sobbed when I finally let myself know that my loved one, as I knew her, is no more. This is one of the hardest life adjustments I have ever made.

331

NOVEMBER 28
Different Milestones

Those of us who have children remember watching for important milestones. We remember the first step, the day that child spoke a sentence, when school started. All these milestones are wonderful memories.

Now we are having to face milestones we never expected to see. Our parent or other loved one needs full-time care. We remember the day we realized their health was really failing. The first time they wet their bed. These are frightening milestones.

It's hard to face our future when it is so uncertain. At least with the children, we knew they would eventually grow up and move away. With our care recipient, it seems they are growing down and moving closer. This is a hard milestone for anyone to handle.

. . . .

These new milestones are hard for me to handle but as I accept the changes I am also accepting my loved one's loss of health. I stand ready to accept whatever comes our way.

Misbehavior

We are not the only ones confused by the change in health. Our care recipient may be just as confused. This is especially true if a brain atrophy disease such as Alzheimer's is the reason for needing a full-time caregiver at home.

There are two unique problems here. The first is that the individual may be frustrated at his inability to do routine tasks, such as making a meal or keeping the check register in order, and he may act out or become depressed.

The second reason, the sadder of the two, is when our loved one becomes aggressive, violent or hard to deal with — perhaps even dangerous to us. If we can no longer handle this, it is time to look for an alternate way such as nursing home or foster home care.

. . . .

I admit to being frightened when my loved one, who in the past wouldn't have hurt an insect, lashes out physically at me all the time. I can no longer give adequate care and I am okay with my decision.

NOVEMBER 30

Nearing The Holidays

With Thanksgiving past, everyone knows that the holidays are drawing near. Every family has established its own holiday traditions. Whatever our religion, or whether we practice a religion at all, we find ourselves drawn into some sort of celebration for the holidays.

Remembering days gone by, we may be in a shopping center, scrambling busily for presents in the few hours we have off. A good suggestion is to shop from catalogs with our care recipient so that both people can participate and enjoy preparing for the holidays.

Having friends, family or other people who are alone over to celebrate in some fashion is a nice way to establish our own brand-new tradition.

....

My life is different now but I need not give away all those things which still are important to me.

No Complaints

It was quite a sight. The daughter was in her 60s, her mother at least 20 years older. The mother was frail and needed assistance with everyday activities; her daughter helped when the mother came to visit from out of town.

The way they looked at each other and cared about each other was priceless. "She never complains," smiled the daughter. Mother and daughter, still a team, even though the daughter was happily married and Mom lived on the other coast with her care attendant.

Willingly, for several months each year, the daughter and her husband did everything they could to make this elderly, graceful woman comfortable. Their mutual caring, respect and strong relationship was beautiful to behold. Many people have wished for such love and caring and were never lucky enough to get it.

. . . .

How special it was to be privileged to see caregiving and love intermingle in such a wonderful warm relationship. I feel joy for that very special mother and her daughter.

DECEMBER 2
Controlling Anger

The situation is common these days. A family member, sometimes a son or daughter, sometimes a spouse, decides to be responsible for the care of an aging, unwell adult. Their intentions are commendable but somewhere between intent and action, a problem develops.

This is most likely to happen if the care recipient no longer can respond to the family member in any lucid way. Unable to follow simple directions or to utter thanks for a well-prepared meal — and the caregiver builds up silent hurt, disappointment and anger until these feelings need an outlet.

Some people can control their anger, talking it out with a friend or counselor or in some other way. With others, it boils over and is released in harsh words or even physical abuse.

. . . .

I was astounded that I hit my wife. At first I cried, then I realized I had to deal with my anger outside the house if I was to continue being her caregiver. The support group has helped immensely.

Self-Imposed Guilt

When we act in an inappropriate way, we suffer guilt. This often happens when a loved one becomes ill and needs to be placed in a nursing home.

Some caregivers just cannot deal with seeing a person they love so much in a care facility, regardless of how lovely it may be. In most cases, the loved one is barely aware of the change in location. Confused and disoriented all the time, that person thinks the nursing home is a nice hotel or hospital and feels pleased to be living there.

The caregiver's guilt is self-imposed; it does not come from the care recipient. After all, we don't place a loved one in a nursing home unless there are no other options.

. . . .

I forgive myself for being human. I recognize that I cannot change the illness; I can only change my own feelings. Knowing how much I care, I absolve myself from guilt.

337

DECEMBER 4

A Fine Experience

Some people take to caregiving very easily while others — willing enough — struggle with each and every day. Taking care of another person's needs is alien and we are not quite sure how to do it and still maintain their dignity.

Learning a new routine is hard, yet many people state that their caregiving has been a wonderful life experience. "I am grateful for the opportunity to pay back all those years she took care of me and our children while I worked," stated one man in the caregiver support group.

Warm and loving, gentle and accepting, these patient and rather unusual folks deeply feel that it is their responsibility and no one else's to care for an elderly loved one. They never make it look hard or inconvenient. They just do their job.

. . . .

This has been an unusual opportunity to pay back the woman who has been my lover, my wife, my helpmate for all our adult life. I enjoy caring for her and will do it as long as necessary.

The inevitable has happened. An invitation has arrived asking us to attend a wedding, a christening, a Bar Mitzvah or an anniversary celebration. We want to go but are unsure how to handle the problem of our care recipient.

There are several solutions. If our care recipient is disruptive or unable to travel, then we might hire someone or ask a family member to take our place while we attend the party alone. Another solution is to take our loved one along with a care attendant. This frees us to enjoy the event.

Consider staying in a motel or hotel rather than with relatives, so that issues which might be embarrassing can be avoided. What matters is that we find a way to get away and attend if it is important to us.

. . . .

The very first time I left my loved one at home with an aide I felt guilty. After that it became easier and now I don't feel so alienated from family and friends. A two-day trip does wonders for me.

339

DECEMBER 6

Intellectualizing

Many people intellectualize their problems, discussing them in a mature and serious way. Attend any support group and we see people who can talk and talk, without getting inside themselves, to express their feelings.

"Well, she has multiple sclerosis, which is a disease where plaque forms . . ." This isn't what the facilitator and other group members want to hear. They want to know how we feel about the fact that our loved one is ill with a progressive disease.

Some never stop intellectualizing but once in a while a caregiver realizes that in order to deal with the situation she needs to express feelings. One man suddenly sobbed out, "You want to know how it feels? I hate that damn disease and what it has done to us!"

....

To my surprise several group members gave me hugs. I finally began to open up the secret place where it hurts me the most. I know sharing will be easier now that I have taken the first step.

Please, Doctor!

"I just can't understand why Dr. Thompson is acting this way. He has taken care of Jimmy for 18 years, from the day he delivered him." Jimmy was dying of leukemia and his mother was confused. She felt that the doctor was pulling away from them.

She may have been right. Some people, even doctors, do not know how to behave when death is approaching. Instead of drawing closer into the circle of support, they move away. What we may not know is that they are hurting, too, and are trying to protect themselves.

Death is never easy. Some people can be supportive and share the pain, cry with us and even sometimes share laughter. Others don't come around because they are protecting themselves or they just don't know what to say.

....

I wish people would understand that just being there helps. Saying "I'm sorry," and not deserting us is what matters. I vow always to be more sensitive to others' needs in times of sorrow.

DECEMBER 8

Friends?

When we have many family members living in the same area, those same family members often are our close friends. Conversely, when we have few or no relatives near by, close friends become just like our family members.

Now we find ourselves in a difficult position. First, we are doing primary caregiving, which is often exhausting and sometimes thankless. Second, our income is likely to have changed, since neither of us can work any longer. Last, we may feel uncomfortable letting our friends know there are financial issues or telling them how hard it is to be on call 24 hours a day.

At this junction we have choices. First, we can let our friends know the truth and invite them into our lives as before, enjoying their friendship. Second, we can be secretive and reclusive and soon our friends will not include us in their activities.

....

The choice is obvious. I need the support and company of my friends and I admit it. Thank goodness for good friends.

DECEMBER 9
Agony And Ecstasy

Pleasure certainly doesn't describe it. Neither does pain or joy. But somewhere among these descriptive words is the experience of caregiving. For each person it is different and each one enters and leaves it differently.

Some days are wonderful, running as smooth as silk, while others are just plain awful. Perhaps these days need to be called the agony and ecstasy of caregiving. As adults, how we do at work reflects what we did when we were younger and how we were brought up. Caregiving does the same, for it, too, is real work.

Hopefully, there will be more good days than bad, more days will be happy than sad. And most important, let's hope that each person treats the other with respect and personal dignity, allowing privacy and time alone.

....

I hope to give my care recipient the best care possible while still being mindful of the need for respect and dignity. And I pray that when I leave this experience, I will feel fulfilled, content and proud.

DECEMBER 10
....
Not A Number

Most of us have heard stories about how people become generic patients when they are in a hospital, not physically lost, but in the never-never land of patienthood. Being in the hospital or very ill is hard enough without also feeling like a number.

The Diabetes In Bed Two, The Stroke In Intensive Care — these are some of the ways that medical professionals may refer to their patients. As caregivers, we need to be extremely careful to stay personal, caring and warm to the person we are caring for so that they do not lose what identity they do have.

The word caregiver implies warmth and caring. Inherent to this job is the importance of treating our care recipient, regardless of his mental state, with respect and understanding.

....

Even when I am angry or overfatigued, I try to remember to treat my care recipient as I would want to be treated. I feel I have done this well.

Telling The Truth

Telling the truth about our loved one, especially if she is either terminally ill or deteriorating mentally, can be extremely difficult and sometimes embarrassing.

Sometimes, when family and friends inquire, it is best to state the facts right away, gently, and then get on with life. Those who care about our recipient deserve to know the truth. Some can take it in one dose while others need to see it unfold over time.

We might need to be careful about telling the whole truth — the brutal truth — if we are talking to people in the presence of our care recipient since they may be shocked, unable or unready to hear it.

....

I respect everyone's right to know the truth and will try to tell it in the way that each can best handle. I am absorbing the truth slowly myself and am letting myself grieve.

DECEMBER 12

Not My Fault

Not all of us have lives which followed a straight and narrow path. Personal problems may have punctuated our adulthood, such as gambling, being abusive or using illegal substances. We may not have always been perfect, and recall that our behavior caused our loved ones grief and pain.

This earlier behavior may come back to haunt us as we caregive for our spouse. Perhaps our loved one has Alzheimer's and is very combative. A spouse who hit that person years before in anger may feel he is only getting his due.

This is sick and convoluted thinking. Behaviors which were out of our control and which have been "fixed" for a long time do not demand retribution and we should not allow it.

....

While I may always feel guilty and sad about my past behavior, I understand that I was ill then. I do not deserve to be treated this way and I know I have to find alternative ways to care for my loved one.

Bouncing Around

Some illnesses are hard to understand, especially those that are characterized by flare-ups and remissions. Multiple sclerosis, lupus, scleroderma and rheumatoid arthritis are a few.

We try our best to caregive for our family member who is having a flare-up. Even though most of us try to continue to work, we still find another full-time job awaiting us at home if our loved one is ill. This is arduous and sometimes confusing since there is no way to know when there will be flare-ups.

Planning ahead becomes almost impossible, and if we do go ahead and make plans, they are likely to be disrupted. Not knowing what tomorrow will bring can cause undue stress in a family. It makes dealing with the illness even more difficult.

....

How selfishly I have been thinking! I have only felt sorry for myself, without realizing how hard it must be to have so much pain and uncertainty in life. I will try much harder to understand.

DECEMBER 14

Hug Me!

One of the first things to go when there is severe illness in the family is physical intimacy. For many reasons, some of which are just not thinking about it, being repelled by the loved one's sick look and fear of hurting the one we love, intimacy gets shoved aside.

This is so sad since so many couples can still touch, kiss or hug each day. Perhaps sex, as we knew it, is out of the question — for now or permanently — but we can still openly show affection, which is needed now more than ever.

When asked what they miss most about their "old life," people may state plaintively, "Sitting next to one another on the couch and watching television," or "Getting a hug when I feel down." Such small requests. Such big problems.

....

We both lost sight of how to touch each other, aside from caregiving needs. Our daily life is better now that we have remembered and are making an effort to be affectionate again.

Blaming God

For some reason, some people have a deep need to find a way to lay blame for their loved one's stroke, accident or illness. While this is not uncommon, it is also not very practical.

Illness and accidents happen and once they have, we can no longer call back good health. We must move on. To spend our day lamenting that it did happen, to spend all our time looking for someone or something to blame it on is a waste of time.

The fact is that our loved one is ill or injured and needs our care. We can decide to give it or have someone else do it but it does need to be done. Now. Today.

....

Putting off the inevitable only puts off my acceptance of what has happened. I will try my best to move on and help all I can.

DECEMBER 16

Depressed Caregivers

At one time or another, almost every family is affected by depression severe enough to need medical treatment. To pretend it doesn't happen is to ignore a highly treatable mental illness. That would be like not taking an infant to the doctor for an ear infection, hoping the infection will go away if we just ignore it.

Care recipients can become depressed and so can caregivers. By sorting out the symptoms that mirror the fatigue and "down" feeling we may experience as caregivers, we will know that something else is going on and we should go for help.

Being depressed and asking for help is not a sign of weakness but of strength instead. Facing up to our physical frailties and admitting we need help is the very first step to recovery.

....

*I was embarrassed to go to the doctor, that
it might look as though I don't have what
it takes to be a good caregiver. Since then,
I have found out how common depression
is and I am happy I went for help.*

Holiday Time

There is no way to deny it. Everywhere we go, whether to a grocery store or a shopping center, evidence is there that holiday time is approaching. The Salvation Army people are ringing bells in every mall and people seem to be scurrying about a bit faster than normal.

Since we can't fight it, we may as well join it! Having some sort of holiday party, even a potluck dinner or just coffee and dessert, we realize that we can actually reconcile taking care of a sick person and giving a small easy party, too.

The people who cared about us before still care and are genuinely happy to spend time with us, especially now that we are a bit more housebound. Friends and family mean everything, especially at this time of year. Friends are meant to enjoy.

. . . .

Many people are lonely at holiday time. We don't need to be among them unless we choose to be.

DECEMBER 18
Changing Rules

In general, morning means that we eat breakfast, noon means lunch and evening's arrival indicates supper. Those are the rules we learned growing up and we stick to them still even though we can make other choices.

Nowadays, unless there is an illness like diabetes or a condition like high cholesterol, we and our care recipient can eat what we want. Maybe cold pizza and a glass of milk sound like a great breakfast. Why not? Who made those rules anyway?

Just so we get our daily quota of all the vitamins and minerals we need, why should it matter if our care recipient wants an ice cream cone and a hard boiled egg for lunch, in that order? Left-over chicken, a plum and a milkshake for breakfast, anyone?

....

Bending the rules has never been my strong point but I understand that so much control has been taken from my loved one that it must feel good to at least have control over something.

Who Am I?

One day Geralynn's mother wandered into her daughter's room during the night. "Who am I?" she wanted to know. Stunned, Geralynn answered, "You're my mother! Beatrice Hugo Bowman." But that wasn't what the elderly and very ill lady wanted to know.

"I used to be a wife, a mother, a grandmother, a friend, a teacher, a volunteer worker and many other things. Who am I now that I am sick? Do I matter to anyone anymore?"

Taking a cue from her mother's question and consternation, Geralynn began making sure that her mother had visitors; she took pictures for a new photo album of her mom with the children, with her and her husband, doing things around the house. She showed her mother that she still had value and that she was very much loved.

. . . .

My mother's sense of worth was destroyed by needing a caregiver. We are all working hard to give her back a sense of dignity and to give her our unwavering support.

DECEMBER 20

Exercising

These days the evidence is everywhere. We are promised we might live longer, look better and feel healthier if only we would exercise daily. Health clubs abound. Joggers and walkers fill the sidewalks near our home in the early morning and evening.

Instead we are stuck at home, caring for a close friend or relative who needs us, not regretting it, but unable to find time to exercise. We begin to cast about for solutions.

One way is to have a neighbor or teenager come in for half an hour daily so we can go for a brisk walk. Another might be to purchase a stationary bike so we can get our exercise without going anywhere. What matters is that we do it.

....

No matter how tired I am each day, I understand how important it is that I exercise. I have worked out a plan with the teenager next door to come in and oversee things so I can go for a walk daily.

354

Not Right

"We used to call it graveyard stew. It was made with warm milk and toast, all mushed together. You just don't do it right," she complained. Poor Herb. He was struggling so hard to help his wife.

Herb knew he was doing his best and that his wife was just frustrated that she could do little but sit in the chair and watch him work. She continually grumbled and he wondered if he were doing a poor job caregiving since she had so many complaints.

What Herb and many other folks just don't realize is that the whole life of some sick people has narrowed to the confines of their house or apartment. They want so badly to feel in control of something that they get in the habit of inadvertently criticizing.

. . . .

I know she loves me and that I am doing a good job but it hurts all the same to be constantly criticized. We will have to talk about how she is hurting me and I will develop thicker armor.

DECEMBER 22
Chore Service

With the double duty of caring for her father and her husband, both in the same home, she hardly had time to go to the bathroom. It got so that the house seemed to be falling down around her.

Errands needed running and all the small repairs her husband always used to do were mounting up. Not knowing where to turn, the woman called a senior service center and they told her about the chore service.

She was informed that teenagers or healthy retired people would come in at very little cost and shovel her walk, mow the lawn, go to the grocery store, maybe even fix the front door screen. She was delighted and relieved to find a service to help her and others.

....

I can't believe there are so many wonderful people willing to go out of their way to help us. The older I get, the nicer people seem to be.

DECEMBER 23
Comfort Stories

Remember when we were small and our parents used to read our favorite stories? *Winnie the Pooh. Alice in Wonderland. The Little Engine That Could. Cinderella. The Just-So Stories.* We cherish and remember those stories even now when we are much older.

Why not reread them, this time aloud, and share with our care recipient? They likely will give just as much comfort and joy as they did when we were children and this time they will provide some entertainment as well.

Children's stories are not just for children. They are for everyone to enjoy. Reading children's books works especially well if our loved one doesn't have a very long span of attention.

. . . .

When this idea was first suggested, I scoffed, but then I tried it. Captivated by Cinderella and my childhood memories, I have read many others aloud. We both enjoy them immensely.

357

DECEMBER 24
A Need To Hide

Constant demands from a sick person who is confused and disoriented are troublesome. We no sooner lie down than we are called again, for our care recipient may no longer have a good sense of time and its passage.

Rarely do we get to eat without cleaning up another spill. Rarely do we ever get to stay in the bathroom as long as we would like to without being called for assistance from the other room. It is so overwhelming that sometimes we feel as though we would like to hide.

When it gets that bad, it is time to either place our loved one in a respite care facility for a day or two to get some time off, consider an adult daycare program or hire a sitter for half a day each week to get away and do whatever we want to do — for ourselves.

....

While I consider myself a patient and careful caregiver, I recognize that I must have some time for myself. I no longer feel guilty taking some time off, for it makes me more relaxed and a better caregiver.

Regardless of our religion — if we practice one — we cannot avoid the fact that this is Christmas day. Turn on the television and there are parades and prayer services on every channel along with multiple showings of *Miracle on 42nd Street*.

Some of us may enjoy this, while others may resent it deeply. Some who are not of the Christian faith wish something else were on television; others may resent it because the programs recall all that we used to do for the holidays.

Perhaps the family went to Midnight Mass or opened one present at midnight. Whatever it was, the tradition is likely to be broken now that we are dealing with ongoing illness and infirmity.

....

What Christmas stands for might still be very important to us but we must celebrate it in our hearts since we cannot do it our old way.

DECEMBER 26
Helping Hands

So many folks — family, friends and some people we barely know — step forward to help in a real crisis. When there is a death in the family or a serious auto accident, helping hands appear out of nowhere to offer solace, to prepare food and to help in other ways.

Unfortunately, our situation isn't a crisis, at least not in the usual sense. What we have is a chronic ongoing need for help. Being the primary caregiver is very hard work and we could use the able assistance of people who care. But no one offers and we don't ask.

It is pride that keeps some people from asking for help and for others it is pure stubbornness. We just don't want anyone to know how bad it is. Until we are willing to admit, at least to ourselves, that we could use some help, no one will offer any.

. . . .

When I finally asked our family for help,
I was amazed how they responded with
offers. How foolish I was to be so proud.

"This was the very first time we had an opportunity to see our brand-new grandchild, a baby girl named Donna. Our son and his wife were bringing her over, along with lunch, that afternoon.

"What excitement, now that I had something to look forward to. Yet my joy was mingled with sadness knowing that my husband would not even recognize our son. Still, I couldn't wait to see their beautiful new baby girl.

"How surprised we all were when Dad — the brand-new grandpa — had a lucid afternoon, billed and cooed over the baby and even held her! What a joy that we could take pictures of that blessed event. Later that night, lucidity passed and confusion returned. But I knew we had witnessed a holiday miracle."

....

Even caregiving has its times of miracles. It really was miraculous that this was a "good day" and everything worked out well.

DECEMBER 28
Bookmobile

Getting to the library is sometimes impossible for a caregiver, especially if it is hard to get our loved one ready to go out. Neighborhood bookmobiles are an answer, for rather than having to go to the library, the bookmobile brings a selection of books to an area near where we live.

The librarian on the bookmobile will, after a while, get to know our taste in books and what we read to our loved one and will bring books, especially if we request them, even bestsellers.

This gives both caregiver and recipient something to look forward to. Books always can help fill quiet times when we need to be doing something for ourselves.

. . . .

Reading is one of my greatest joys and I am so happy that I can get to the bookmobile to stock up on reading material.

Regardless of the age we are, unless we are in the child-raising years, it seems everyone enjoys watching young children while they play. They are cute and funny.

Going into a restaurant, we may be surprised to see how much our care recipient, regardless of his level of functioning, likes watching people, particularly small children.

We might decide, then and there, to make it a point to go out more often together. It is a nuisance sometimes, to get everything in place for an excursion, so we tend not to go.

. . . .

I hadn't realized that we were staying at home because it was too much trouble for me to get things ready. I will no longer do that; it is not fair to my loved one.

Overview

Now another whole year has gone by. It was filled with joys and sorrow. Caregiving is like that, full of joy, sorrow, sadness, anticipation and hope.

Hope stays alive, as we never give up wishing that things will improve for our loved one, that there will be a new medicine to help or some magic surgery to cure our loved one. Everyone needs to have something to hope for.

By and large, most of us are proud that we have made it successfully through another whole year. We feel a tremendous sense of pride in the difficult job we are doing.

....

As long as I can continue to hope, I can continue to caregive.

New Year's Eve

Memories of years gone by filter through our mind on this last day of the year. Remember all the good parties we went to and how much fun we had screaming "Happy New Year!" at the stroke of midnight?

Now our life has done a full turnaround. An individual we have loved for all these years, a wife, husband, parent, sibling or child is ill. We are the primary caregiver, something we never could have conceived of when we were young. The old days are gone forever.

But the new days are here right now. Rather than lamenting what we no longer have, we can use this time to find those things we can still be thankful for. Our own good health. The fact that our loved one is still alive. Our family and friends. Perhaps our outside job.

....

There is always something to look forward to and there are always people worse off than we are. I am grateful we have this time to be together and that I am able to openly show my love and caring.

Best Sellers From HCI

ISBN	TITLE	PRICE
1-55874-112-7	Adult Children of Alcoholics (Expanded)	$8.95
0-932194-54-0	Bradshaw On: The Family	$9.95
0-932194-26-5	Choicemaking	$9.95
1-55874-040-6	Perfect Daughters	$8.95
1-55874-105-4	The Laundry List	$9.95
0-932194-40-0	Healing The Child Within	$8.95
0-932194-39-7	Learning To Love Yourself	$7.95
0-932194-25-7	Struggle For Intimacy	$6.95
0-932194-68-0	Twelve Steps To Self-Parenting For Adult Children	$7.95

Orders must be prepaid by check, money order, MasterCard or Visa. Purchase orders from agencies accepted (attach P.O. documentation) for billing. Net 30 days.

TOTAL ORDER VALUE	ADD
$0 - 10.00	$3.00
$10.01 - 25.00	$4.00
$25.01 - 50.00	$4.50
Orders over $50.00 in the U.S.	9%
Orders over $50.00 outside U.S.	15%

* Shipping prices subject to change without prior notice.

Health Communications, Inc.
3201 S.W. 15th Street
Deerfield Beach, FL 33442-8190
(800) 851-9100